Facebuilder FOR MEN

Facebuilder FOR MEN

Carole Maggio & Mike Gianelli

A fast, effective, and proven
muscle-toning program

A PERIGEE BOOK

A Perigee Book
Published by The Berkley Publishing Group
A division of Penguin Putnam Inc.
375 Hudson Street
New York, New York 10014

Previously published in Great Britain by Pan Books
First Perigee edition: July 2002

Perigee ISBN: 0-399-52784-2

Visit our website at www.penguinputnam.com

This book has been catalogued with the Library of Congress.

Printed in the United States of America

10 9 8 7 6 5 4 3 2 1

CONTENTS

This book is dedicated to Matthew Sanchez, whose determination and dedication to facial improvement have been a major inspiration to me. I am grateful for his vision, support and encouragement. To Jeff and Brit, two young men who have helped me stay young at heart and who have made me realize that you're never too young to start caring about how you look and feel. To Keith, who kept my computer up and running day and night, and who taught me not to crash and burn when my hard drive did. To Linda Bollman and CoValence, Inc. for all their cutting-edge antiaging information. And to M.G., who, at sixty-one years old, is the epitome of grace, elegance and charm and who is my male role model.

INTRODUCTION

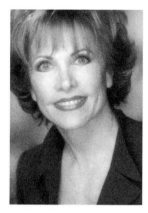

Facebuilder for Men is exactly what the name implies. Everyone knows that you can build and define your body by exercising. No secret there. What many don't know is that you can do the same thing for your face. That's been a big secret for a long time.

A defined face requires toned, taut muscles under the skin. To achieve this, you need to exercise the muscles of the face. The good news here is that since the muscles of the face are smaller than most other muscles in the body, they respond much more quickly to exercise.

Facebuilder is an easy-to-do facial exercise regime which will definitely assist you in building a firm, strong jawline, a taut, toned face and an overall younger appearance. If you are willing to invest the ten minutes a day it takes to achieve that younger look you desire and deserve, you'll get that look and keep it indefinitely.

When you finish reading this book, you will have all the tools it takes to go to work on your face and you'll see very positive results very quickly. It's quick, simple and, best of all, it works like a charm.

The famous baseball pitcher Satchel Page once said, "Age is a question of mind over matter. If you don't mind, it don't matter." Does looking and feeling older than you are matter to you? If it does, then this exercise program is what you've been looking for. Doing the Facebuilder exercises for ten minutes a day is all it takes to turn back the clock and postpone Father Time's inexorable march across your face. They say that Time marches on. With Facebuilder, it doesn't have to march on over you.

1

Build your Face

I've always felt that looking good makes you feel good. However, it requires work and the hectic lifestyle most men have today doesn't allow much time for anything other than their careers. Many men simply don't have the time to squeeze in an exercise program, even though they know they should. And it gets worse the older they become. As American poet Robert Frost said, "By working faithfully eight hours a day, you may eventually get to be a boss and work twelve hours a day."

Facebuilder is a natural answer, however. It's perfect if you're busy, whether or not you're the boss. It'll only take ten minutes a day for you to develop a tight, youthful face—and you don't need props, machines, a gym, or tools of any kind to do these exercises. You were born with the only tools you'll ever need to exercise the fifty-seven muscles of your face.

Why appearance matters

We all know that exercise is necessary to maintain a good-looking body, but most people don't think about keeping their faces in shape, even though this part of them is much more on view than any other. You'd think in a society that puts as much emphasis on facial appearance as ours does, proper facial care would be a top priority, but it isn't. And that is particularly true for men. The last part of their bodies most men think about keeping in shape is their faces, but they are having to rethink their attitudes and their ideas are being dragged, kicking and screaming, into the twenty-first century. Today, it's important to look as good as you can. It's a youthful marketplace out there and fiercely competitive. How you look sells you to the public, your boss and to your clients, not to mention to the ladies. Like it or not, society places a very high premium on looking youthful and fit. It may not seem fair, but life is not always fair. As Johnny Carson once said, "If life were fair, Elvis would be alive and all the impersonators would be dead."

We are inexorably attracted to attractive things and not to be aware of this is to overlook a fundamental basic of life. Not sure about that? Then let me give you a little bit of information to reinforce that statement. Statistics show that approximately 95 percent of all adults place a very high premium on facial appearance when evaluating another person. First impressions are *very* important. It's a fact that you never get a second chance to make a good first impression. Also, a recent survey of many women showed that they preferred a man to have a youthful face rather than a muscular body. Surprised? You shouldn't be. Most women are *much* less impressed with muscle than you think.

Recently, while working out in a gym in my home town, I struck up a conversation with a lady on the treadmill next to me. As we walked off a few calories (probably three or four), she said to me, while looking around the room, "It's a shame that so many of the men in here have such young-looking bodies but they don't have young-looking faces." She was right. Men may want good-looking bodies, and they may want their partners to have good-looking bodies, but women don't focus on the same things. Girls want their guys to look youthful. Ever since I was a teenager, I would notice a guy's face first. To be sure, there were lots of hunks around, especially in high school and at college, and you couldn't help noticing their physiques, because they were right in your face. You could almost smell the testosterone, but that didn't impress my friends or me. We liked nice-looking faces. We still do.

Most of the men I know now say that they can pretty easily cover up their shortcomings with the right clothes and it helps if they have a nice set of wheels, but they can't do much about their facial imperfections. Clothes don't address that. Facial exercises do. Facebuilder is the key to working on your face and making the positive changes you want to see.

Your face comes first

Women long ago realized how important their facial appearance was. Great makeup, skincare and hairstyles have worked magic for women for centuries. Cleopatra didn't charm Julius Caesar and Mark Antony with her figure. In fact history books refer to her as being somewhat overweight and frumpy. That didn't stop her because she was clearly seductive. She was a real pro when it came to makeup and looking as good as she could with the somewhat limited features God (or Ra) gave her. She had access to the best makeup ingredients ancient Egyptian alchemists could devise. And it worked, didn't it? Julius and Mark were drawn to her because of the way she looked.

The face of another woman, Helen of Troy, was so beautiful it was rumored to have "launched a thousand Greek ships" resulting in a ten-year war between the Greeks and the Trojans. Now *that's* what I call a beautiful face.

Recent statistics indicate that guys are finally noticing the importance of looking their best. For example, one out of three surgical procedures performed by plastic surgeons are now on men. That's a truly huge leap from just a few years ago when most or all of the procedures were on women. In addition, more and more men are entering bastions of beauty that were previously a women-only zone. The reason is probably that men are finally realizing that their faces are as important as their resumes. The guys know that they need to look fresh and alert, not tired and drawn, if they are to be taken seriously in the workplace, or in any place for that matter.

It was recently reported that between 1996 and 2001 the world market for male cosmetics and beauty products had grown by nearly 40 percent. It's huge now and will just keep getting bigger each year. More and more men are going to beauty salons for facials, massages and aromatherapy. There is a wide range of other treatments available now too, such as teeth whitening, hair transplants, laser-eye surgery to eliminate glasses, laser-hair removal, testosterone replacement and antiaging treatments. One of the top six non-surgical rejuvenation techniques being offered by plastic surgeons' clinics today is customized exercise programs, which should include facial exercises. The "make myself look better" syndrome just keeps on truckin'. It all goes to show that men are now as interested in how they look as women always have been. It looks like Mae West was right when she exclaimed, "Too much of a good thing is a good thing."

The background to Facebuilder

For years, I had been aware that men wanted to have better facial appearances (whether you guys would admit it or not), but my focus had, until recently, been directed towards the ladies. In 1995, I published *Facercise*, a book on facial exercises. It has been a bestseller for years and I have recently brought out a new edition, which includes additional exercises.

During the years I've been teaching facial exercises, I've acquired a very extensive knowledge of how different faces age. I've also learned how they can be successfully toned, sculpted and firmed by exercising the facial muscles. I've given seminars and classes all over the world, working on people with all types of skin, facial shapes and problems unique to themselves, including Bell's palsy, temporomandibular joint syndrome (TMJ) and other facial irregularities caused by genetics, disease and accidents. I know now that every face, regardless of age, sex, shape or texture, can derive antiaging benefits from a personalized facial exercise program.

Facercise has become a worldwide phenomenon and has been named one of the top one hundred beauty products in the world. I've worked with socialites, rock stars, royalty, celebrities of every type, politicians, athletes and business leaders from all walks of life. Over the last few years, I've received numerous requests from men for an exercise program, so I decided that this would be the ideal time to introduce *Facebuilder for Men*. I've seen, from personal experience, the dramatic change men can achieve by doing these exercises. Facebuilder will help create a rejuvenated face for any guy who is interested in gaining and maintaining that competitive edge.

The concept of Facebuilder started evolving several years ago after I face-trained Anthony, an attractive executive who worked for a giant computer company in California's Silicon Valley. He was a tall, distinguished man who looked older than his fifty-eight years. Before we started his three-day exercise session, he told me that he had tried everything he could to keep in shape. "Carole," he said, "I work out in the gym daily. I eat right. But no matter how much iron I pump or how many marathons I run, I don't look like the younger employees I oversee." He had a large staff of young people working for him and he liked to call them "the kids." "I feel like the old man around the office," he said, "I don't want to look like an old dude or be perceived as old by the kids." He wanted to be on the cutting edge and he didn't feel that the "old guys" were perceived to possess that edge. In short, he wanted to turn back the clock. He mentioned that if you were in your twenties or thirties, you could be scruffy *and* cool, but not in your fifties. His bottom line was, "I've got to compete in a business world full of young people and I want to look like I belong in that world." He felt, at fifty-eight, that he had to look better and that was becoming increasingly difficult because he felt his skin and his body was starting to fall apart. He would have agreed with Darrick Antell, M.D., a top New York plastic surgeon, who said, "In America, people's consciousness of looks is quite high because importance is attached to appearance in a business situation."

I took "before" and "after" pictures of Anthony and I showed him the pictures at the end of the third day. He looked at the "before" picture, gasped and said, "I didn't know I had such a prominent double chin." Then he looked at the second picture. He was absolutely amazed at the difference he saw in his chin and jawline. They were more toned and defined. His eyes had a more rested, open appearance. His gray pallor had changed to a more healthy-looking color. In a nutshell, he looked like he had just spent three weeks playing golf at his favorite resort. He was totally enthused with his new look. "I'm doing these exercises forever," he told me. I still get a call or a card from him now and then. The last card was a cute one. It said, "I don't look like the old dude any more. I look like the lead dog now." I got a kick out of that, especially since only the lead dog has a change of scenery.

The second motivating factor for putting together the Facebuilder program was the progress made by Matthew, a young man whom I had never met. He emailed me to say how amazed he was with his facial exercise program. He had purchased my book and had been doing the exercises for around a year. He was so impressed with his progress that he had put up a website to exhibit his facial changes. When I viewed his website pictures, I was totally blown away at the positive changes he had made. You *can* see "before" and "after" pictures of Matthew on page 33. You'll be amazed, too.

The transformation of these two people, plus the myriad requests I've had from men wanting specific exercises for their faces, have led me to create Facebuilder, the ultimate face exercise program designed specifically for men. It's a competitive world out there. As Anthony, my business client told me, "You want to be the lead dog." This program will give you the edge you need (and deserve) to get to the top. You *can* change the way you look. Don't be the guy to whom Groucho Marx was referring when he said, "I never forget a face but, in your case, I'll be glad to make an exception."

Why surgery isn't always the best option

When you exercise your face, you are also relieving stress and tension, allowing the muscles to relax. This combats the formation of those question mark and worry lines we all acquire. These lines, over time, have a detrimental effect on the face, which is why more and more men are electing to go under the knife to alleviate these tell-tale signs of aging.

As my business has expanded, I have seen and worked with thousands of clients who have elected to have plastic surgery. I've seen positive and negative results. Successful plastic surgery can rejuvenate your appearance and improve your self-image and confidence. However, plastic surgery is not the right solution for everyone. There can be drawbacks. For example, it is more difficult to get a good result if you're male. Male facial skin has a richer blood supply than female facial skin so male faces bleed more during surgery and are at greater risk of haematomas (a collection or pooling of blood under the skin). Scarring, which may result from surgery, is more difficult for men to camouflage since they don't normally use makeup or style their hair towards their faces as women can do. They also have to contend with abnormal hair and beard growth after a facelift. If hair-growing skin from the upper neck is pulled up behind the ears during surgery, the man will then have to shave behind the ears (which was disastrous for Vincent Van Gogh) or shave the back of the neck (and you thought ordinary shaving was a drag). Men usually end up needing electrolysis or a stint under the laser to get rid of the relocated hair. When that happens they know the kind of hassle women go through to look good for them. Payback time!

Moreover, the results of plastic surgery are fleeting. The beneficial effects of the average facelift last around five to seven years. Going back for seconds will not necessarily give the same results. The reasons for this are numerous: the skin is more brittle and has less elasticity, for example, and the fat has diminished under the facial skin. In addition, the muscles atrophy with age.

This aging process is a gift from our non-genetic parents, Mother Nature and Father Time and it happens to all of us, whether we've had any cosmetic surgery or not. I like to call this nature's double whammy. Although it's definitely a fact that surgery can pull the skin tight across the face, the elements that caused the wrinkles and sags are still inexorably at work. In time, these factors will result in the same wrinkles and sags, evident before the facelift, to start reappearing.

These formidable odds obviously don't deter some of the biggest names in Hollywood, however. If you want to see for yourself how some of these procedures turned out, have what I call a "fright night." Go to see some recent movies featuring some of yesterday's biggest male actors who have now gone under the knife. There's at least a baker's dozen of them out there. It's not a pretty picture. More like a Rocky Mountain Horror Show. And remember, these guys have lots of cash and the surgeons whom they selected were the *very best that money could buy.* Yikes. It brings to mind an interview in the *Los Angeles Times* with John Cleese from the comedy program *Monty Python's Flying Circus*, who was filming a BBC documentary called *The Human Face with John Cleese.* He was asked why people's appearances often change so radically after plastic surgery. He answered that he was horrified at the results some very well-known men, whom he didn't want to name in print, had experienced. He said, "It was obvious that the surgery had quite clearly gone wrong." He probably had a "fright night" of his own. The purpose of Facebuilder is to educate you guys so that you don't ever have to have a first facelift, much less a second one. You don't want to star in your own "fright night," do you?

Think about Robert Redford's wise words. He said, "I'm not a face-lift person. I just don't want to do it . . . for me, the trade-off is that something of your soul in your face goes away . . . You end up looking body-snatched in the last analysis."

Cosmetic surgery also is not a cheap option. More than 60 percent of my clients are people who have had elective plastic surgery of some type or another. They've undergone blepharoplasty (eyelift), a rhinoplasty (nose job) or a complete face-lift. According to the American Society of Plastic Surgeons, more than one million men (an all-time record) had surgical or non-surgical cosmetic procedures in the year 2000. The top five male procedures are eyelid surgery, liposuction, nose reshaping, breast reduction (to correct the effects of gynaecomastia, a condition caused by hormonal abnormality) and facelifts. None of these procedures are inexpensive, either. The average fee for eyelid surgery (both upper and lower) is $3000. The average fee for a face-lift, not including the eyes, is $5500, and that fee does not include the anaesthetic (mandatory, unless you're really into pain) and any other related expenses. As for the costs of liposuction, the average price is around $1900 per site, and most guys have plenty of sites for the surgeon and his cannula to visit. And a man's "boob job" isn't a cheapie, either. If you plan on getting any of these procedures, be ready to launch a serious assault on your IRA and other saving plans. These prices will definitely give a new meaning to the word "ouch."

Alternative to surgery

I can empathize with people who have suffered a botched operation. When I had a nose job at the age of twenty-two I ended up with a dent on one side of my nose and the tip of my nose appeared to be too long. I had spent good money for the procedure, experienced some pain and inconvenience while I recuperated, and I ended up with a nose that did not make me happy. I felt it was definitely less attractive after I underwent the surgery. I have to admit that I shed a few tears over how my operation had turned out and to say that I was rather disappointed would have been a major understatement. However, after I had developed the Facercise exercises, and did them religiously in the course of several months, I was able to shorten my nose tip and fill out the dent. So, the good news is, even if you've gone under the knife, you can still benefit from doing the Facebuilder exercises because they will keep your muscles toned and your skin looking supple. Practicing the Facebuilder techniques guarantee that you will *never* have to shave behind your ears, go under the electric needle or visit your nearest laser center. You can achieve the same results without the drawbacks of surgery and the cost is a microscopic fraction of what a plastic surgeon would charge. As one of America's founding fathers Ben Franklin once said, "an ounce of prevention is worth a pound of cure."

While I am not opposed to plastic surgery, it's extremely important to know that there is always an element of risk, medical and psychological, inherent in such procedures. No reputable plastic surgeon will guarantee to deliver positive results to each and every patient on whom they perform these operations. As I've mentioned previously, health, age and the elasticity of the skin all play a large part in the overall outcome of the procedure. There are numerous factors to be weighed up, which do not come into play if you take the non-surgical route and try facial exercises. What's more, there are many enlightened doctors who value skincare treatments and facial exercises as important adjuncts to surgery. I've had plastic surgeons refer their patients to me because they know that facial exercises can help reshape muscles weakened from atrophy, accidents, facelifts and surgical modifications. Dr. Lawrence Birnbaum, a well-known Beverly Hills plastic surgeon, in a letter to me, stated that "in my instructions to patients, I frequently encourage them to do facial exercises."

I would sum it up as saying Facebuilder is like going to the gym on a regular basis. If you work out at the gym, you *know* you are going to see favorable results. It's the same with Facebuilder: You make the effort, your face reaps the rewards.

My clients I mentioned earlier that I receive many, many letters from clients, some of whom are men. I would like to share with you some of the comments from these guys.

Ben Dickson, a twenty-eight-year-old from Phoenix, writes, "I had a nose, which I'd broken years ago in a football game. While some people said it gave me character, I didn't see it that way. I saw your exercises in a book my girlfriend was reading and I had her show me the nose exercise, which I did for several weeks. I noticed a difference in the symmetry and shape and I've been doing them ever since."

≡ Ron Gardner, thirty-two, from Boston, says, "Everyone said I looked like Rocky, because my eyes looked sleepy. I saw you on TV, talking about your book, so I bought it and did the eye exercises. I was amazed at the change. It was definitely an 'eye-opening' experience. No one is calling me Rocky now."

≡ Dan Gaylord, sixty, from Los Angeles writes, "I'm in sales and I have to address clients who are much younger on a daily basis. I sell vitamins and I discovered your book in a healthfood shop. I was always a little embarrassed at how I looked lately because I was looking older than my age. I felt the younger clients would doubt the benefit of what I was selling because of my age and my appearance. Since I've been doing the exercises, I think I look great. I've even had compliments from the younger clients. Things like, 'You sure don't look your age.' It's music to my ears."

≡ Dan Anderson, a twenty-eight-year-old from New York writes, "I am a musician and keeping my mouth muscles strong gives me a longer career in music. Your exercises have enabled me to maintain a purity of sound and resonance on my trombone."

Some of my correspondents talk about accidents and congenital defects, which have caused facial deformities. I am always amazed when I read how some of my clients rehabilitate themselves with the exercises.

≡ Ian Weeler, a seventy-two-year-old from Germany wrote, "I had major reconstructive jaw surgery on my upper and lower jaw to correct a severe misalignment. The surgery was 'muscle invasive.' As swelling goes away, you are left with sagging facial muscles that have forgotten what to do. They took six inches of bone out of my face, which left me with excessive skin, which needed to be toned up. With your exercises, I'm gaining control of my muscles once again and everything is moving back where it belongs instead of falling down to my neck."

▣ Tom Zane, a twenty-one-year-old from Dallas said, "I was hit by an eighteen-wheeler truck and had five bones in my face broken. Your exercises relieved the numbness and coldness in my face."

▣ Jimmy Goodman, a fifty-eight-year-old from Australia wrote to me to say, "I suffered a bad whiplash injury when someone rear-ended me. I saw chiropractors, acupuncturists, medical doctors, everything. Nothing they did made my pain go away. I tried your exercises at the suggestion of my family doctor as a last resort and, after a month, I could move around like I used to. The pain is virtually all gone. If I hadn't experienced this myself, I never, ever would have believed it. You should be a doctor and your book should be in a medical library."

▣ Dennis Rouck, a thirty-six-year-old college professor from San Francisco wrote, "I've been afflicted with Bell's palsy for over a year. One side of my face looked weak and tired. I've tried many suggestions from doctors to alleviate the effects, but to no avail. My sister gave me a copy of your book because there was a reference in there to my problem. I started doing your exercises and within a month the weak side of my face was stronger and more toned and I had regained the natural symmetry of my face."

Benefits of Facebuilder

The above comments from my clients show that there are reasons to do facial exercises that go far beyond improving your looks. There are excellent therapeutic and restorative benefits that transcend the usual reasons for exercising your face. I continually stress these benefits to my clients. It's as clear as a bell to me. Facial exercises definitely work and they even sometimes perform miracles. It always astounds me when I read an article or an interview by someone in the medical profession who states empirically that there is no scientific evidence that facial exercises work. I wish they would say that with a straight face to my millions of satisfied clients who know from experience the absurdity of that kind of statement. Let them make those statements to Dr. Wilma Bergfeld M.D., a past president of the American Academy of Dermatology, who stated "those who call exercising facial muscles heresy aren't using the available medical knowledge about the effect on overlying structure when you make muscles larger."

On that subject, I can still vividly remember watching Jack LaLanne, America's first body fitness guru, talking about face and body exercises on his TV shows in the 1950s. While other kids were watching *Flash Gordon*, I was watching Jack's exercise programs. Even back then, as a young girl, I was in agreement with his philosophy regarding exercise. It made absolute sense to me then, just as it does now. On his website, Jack states, "I was forty years ahead of my time. The doctors were against me, but I knew more about the workings of the muscles in my body than most doctors." Jack's eighty-seven at the time of writing and he looks great. The medical profession hammered him unmercifully all those years ago, ridiculing him and stating that there was no scientific evidence that exercising the muscles of the body really worked. Really! Those who criticize facial exercises, whether in the medical profession or the media, remind me of a comment made by Christopher Morley. He said, "A critic is a gong at the railway crossing, clanging loudly and vainly as the train rolls by." Chris, my man, I couldn't have put it better myself.

Many in the medical field are more enlightened, however. Dr. Gerald Walman, an Arizona ocular plastic surgeon said, "Facercise is a carefully researched and scientifically developed method of exercising individual facial muscles and sets of muscles. I saw that these exercises can and do effect positive changes in tightening and firming the upper and lower eyelids." And Beverly Hills plastic surgeon Dr. Lawrence Birnbaum has stated that, "logic seems to dictate that good facial exercises would prevent many of the aging manifestations." When Dr. Wilma Bergfield, head of dermatology in the Department of Pathology at the Cleveland Clinic Foundation, was being interviewed by the magazine *Vogue*, she was asked what could be done to stop sagging facial muscles. Her response was, "exercise." Finally in the book *Prescription for Nutritional Health, America's Number 1 Guide to Natural Health*, the authors recommend "exercise your face" to combat wrinkles. There you have it, guys. That puts the ball in your court now, doesn't it?

Benefits for you

Facebuilder is the most user-friendly facial exercise program ever invented. You can do the exercises anywhere, anytime. Consider this book your personal trainer for facial fitness. Take pictures of yourself, both front and profile shots and then repeat this in fourteen days. Use the same pose, clothes and lighting. Don't smile in either set of photos. You be the judge of the results. For about the price of a movie and a Coke and ten minutes of your time a day, you'll achieve positive facial changes you never thought possible. And remember that pictures don't lie. Your friends might, but not your camera.

Facebuilder will counteract gravity's insidiously constant pull on your face. You are in control. Each day you will be able to see how you are making progress in holding the aging process at bay. You *can* turn back the clock and slow down the inexorable hands of time. But you do have to make an effort and stick with the program. Remember, as the economist Milton Friedman said, "there's no such thing as a free lunch."

Regarding the human face, there's some good news and some bad news, which needs to be illuminated here.

The bad news as your face ages

■ Your skin starts to look gray and sallow

■ The nose continues to grow longer and wider

■ Eyelids and eyebrows start to droop

■ Under-eye puffiness increases

■ The jawline starts to sag

■ Jowls develop

■ A double chin starts to form

The good news as you Facebuild

■ Your skin becomes more healthy-looking

■ The nose will start to shorten and narrow

■ The eyelids and eyebrows raise

■ The under-eye puffiness starts to diminish

■ The jawline firms up

■ The jowls tone and tighten

■ The double chin recedes

I can tell you, without reservation, that if you do Facebuilder exercises properly, you will see and feel tremendous changes in your face as well as an elevation in self-esteem. These changes will improve your face, enhance your life and give you a leg up in the competitive business world.

2

How Facebuilder works

Good bone structure, a sculpted, firm jawline, a well-shaped nose and youthful-looking eyes are all facial features most of us wish we had. Most people would credit good bone structure as the key component of facial attractiveness, but few people realize what an important role muscles play in moulding the contours of the face. Without facial muscles, we couldn't blink, smile or frown. The face would be just a mask, nothing more. Since the muscles in the face are smaller and thinner than most other muscles in the body, they respond more quickly to an exercise regime. Because the fat-to-muscle ratio in the face is lower than it is in most other parts of the body, the effects of facial exercises are visible in a very short period of time.

Some muscles in our bodies get exercised whether or not we mean intentionally to exercise them. We don't voluntarily have to exercise our legs, arms or hands, for example. They are active from the time we climb out of bed and they continue to be exercised until we go to bed. We don't use our facial muscles in quite the same fashion. These muscles need specific exercises if we want to develop them and make them look as good as they should. Picture the stomach of someone who never works out.

Not a pretty picture, is it? Now picture that same stomach on someone who exercises that area consistently. Is there any difference between the two in your mind? <u>Abs</u>olutely.

The same concept applies to our faces. We don't have to like it but we all subconsciously know that when muscles sag, the skin attached to the muscles also sags. Slack facial muscles are the primary cause of the sagging, the drooping, the bags under the eyes, the pouches and the unsightly jowls many of us develop as we get older. Lack of the proper facial exercise allows the muscle tissue to become thin and atrophied. This results in a person looking old. Remember the George Burns comment that "you don't have to be old to look old"? That's right on the money.

Working the facial muscles

There is a viable alternative to looking old, however, and I'm sharing it with you in Facebuilder. Isolating and working the muscles in the face to the point of feeling a lactic acid burn is the key to why Facebuilder works so efficiently. This tingling, burning sensation occurs when a muscle is worked to capacity. The muscle produces lactic acid as a result of the expenditure of energy. It has used up its ATP (adenosine triphosphate), a nucleotide present in all living cells that is vital to energy production. Exercise physiologists and personal trainers are very familiar with this energy burning process. They refer to ATP as "the energy molecule." That, in a nutshell, explains the lactic burn. Experiencing this burn lets you know that you are making the muscle stronger and larger. This process restores the muscle tissue, elasticity and tone, resulting in plump, stronger facial muscles. It's your body telling you you're making progress.

Muscles are fibrous masses of tissues, which are comprised of protein. Exercising these muscles promotes the thickening and strengthening of the muscle fibers. To make a muscle stronger, there must be adequate amounts of protein in the diet to ensure muscle growth. Red meat, fish, chicken, turkey and eggs are tremendous sources of protein and they are easily accessible. Make sure you eat some protein with each meal. (See also Good Nutrition, p. 86.)

You need to work your muscles until they tire to ensure the maximum results. Tennis ace Jimmy Connors knew what he was talking about when he said, "Use it or lose it." The more a muscle contracts, the more it grows. It is also important to remember that after the muscle tires, rest is absolutely essential. This allows the muscle tissue to regenerate and grow larger and stronger. With the right balance of exercise, rest and protein, the muscles adapt to the demands placed on them, producing beneficial results. By isolating facial muscles and performing repeated exercises, the muscles are strengthened, regenerated and toned. You guys all know this regime works on your body muscles from your gym days. Well, it works with facial muscles, too. You just don't have to go to the gym to achieve facial muscle development.

Facebuilder will teach you eleven facial exercises which will isolate and work the fifty-seven muscles in the face and neck area. The face and neck muscles are interconnected by an intricate network of fibers and these exercises ensure that every muscle benefits from the workout.

What to Expect from Facebuilder

Facebuilder will educate you on how facial muscles work. You'll learn to isolate the specific muscle groups in your face. You'll also learn that these exercises can be performed while doing normal day-to-day activities. Facial exercises can be done while you are lying in bed before you get up in the morning, showering, while driving your car to work, working on your computer, etc. You'll also learn that there are no "quick fix" methods to arrive at the results you will want.

Everyone knows that the key to building body muscle is multiple sets of repetitions. Facebuilder is the first facial exercise program that applies the same principles for facial muscles. You have to work the program consistently, making this a part of your daily routine. Muscles are lazy, like many people. They only do what they have to do, nothing more. You need to take charge here. Be the Boss. Make them work for you.

In these health-conscious times, most of us are aware of what we need to do if we want to build muscle and reduce body fat. A low-fat diet, regular aerobic exercise and a carefully devised weight-training program are the ticket here. No short cuts will work effectively over the long haul. Face exercises need to become a daily routine as basic as getting up in the morning, going to work and going to bed at night.

The benefits of Facebuilder

Ever since I started teaching face exercises, I have continuously consulted plastic surgeons, dermatologists and physical therapists to constantly refine the exercises and make sure they are as effective and current as possible. I've been asked, on numerous occasions, whether facial exercises will deepen wrinkles, or stretch out your skin. Actually, just the opposite occurs. As you exercise, you increase the blood circulation to the muscles and other areas of the face. This results in firmer muscles, better blood circulation and color to the face and tauter skin. The skin smooths out and the wrinkles become less visible. These exercises will greatly improve your skin tone from the inside, unlike plastic surgery. And without the ouch.

One of the key reasons Facebuilder is so effective is that it combines two of our most readily renewable assets: visualization and the energy to focus. Your ability to visualize your muscles expanding and building and your energy to focus on specific muscle groups plays a crucial role in making Facebuilder work effectively. I like to call it the "mind-muscle" connection. When I am coaching my clients, I tell them that they must feel their muscles working and I stress that they need to visualize their muscles expanding with every repetition. As you do the Facebuilder techniques you will learn to recognize the burning sensation in the facial muscles as an indication that you are doing the exercises correctly. With such a powerful physical feeling on which to focus, your mind stays honed, tuned in and on track, and you can actually feel the muscles expand as you work towards achieving your goals. Your thoughts are equally as powerful as your actions because you are feeling your muscles expand and strengthen as you progress. Your reward for this effort is the youthful, toned, defined face you deserve. When George Orwell said, "By the age of fifty, every man has the face he deserves," he obviously was not aware of Facebuilder.

Clients have told me that one of the most exciting moments to occur, after they have started face exercises, is when they actually start to *feel* the muscles in their faces. They become conscious of that usually "dead" area between the cheekbones and mouth or the space between the ear and the nose. It's similar to the feeling you get in your arms or legs when you start up an exercise program. You can tell something is different. You might feel a little sore but it's a good ache because you instinctively know that you've really worked those muscles and they're aching and rebuilding at the same time. Incidentally, when you're exercising your facial muscles and you feel that lactic acid burn, I suggest alleviating the burn feeling by blowing out through your closed lips. This will release the stored lactic acid in the muscle, just the same as stretching leg or arm muscles feel better after you've exercised those areas. When my clients feel those muscles working, they are encouraged because they can tell that the exercises are working. You will be, too.

I'm extremely proud to be able to offer people such a healthy, easy, effective program to improve their facial appearance. Facebuilder is effective for numerous reasons and one of them is that the techniques are so easy to master. We all make faces throughout the day. Now, with Facebuilder, you are going to learn how to make faces that will be beneficial, not detrimental, to your face. Also, the exercises are very effective stress-busters, which relax your face, body and mind. Are there any other benefits? Well, you don't need props, gimmicks, gloves or any special place to do them. Need any more reasons? How about looking so good that girls start asking you out—and offer to pay? Now, that's a really cool benefit, wouldn't you say?

3

Let's face facts

How to pinpoint and understand your unique
facial features

OK, guys, time to get serious and buckle down. We've already seen how important your looks are to other people. Dr. Joyce Brothers, in her *US* magazine column, stated that "if you're attractive, people are much more likely to remember whatever it is you are saying. How a person looks, no matter what their age, is always important and physical attractiveness matters the most in initial or one-time encounters." When you're out and about in the business world, meeting people and selling yourself, you need to keep this in mind. Always remember how important first impressions are. That's never been more true than it is in today's competitive arena. It's a rat race out there and, apparently, the most attractive rats are the winners.

The self-image of most people is inexorably tied to their physical appearance. When you were growing up, you wanted to be bigger and stronger than the next boy. You also probably wanted to be better looking. What's the status of your self-image now? How do you really feel about your appearance? Be honest here. There are probably some features that you do like. But aren't there also some features you don't like or would like to change? Virtually no one has perfect features. Heredity plays a large part in how we turn out. We also know that features can be altered surgically and many men seem to be going down that road. Are you prepared to go under the knife to get the look you want (another definition of cutting edge)? You can, of course, but plastic surgery doesn't come with a money-back guarantee if it fails to measure up to your pre-surgery expectations. There is a viable alternative to the anaesthetic and the scalpel. And it's not going to hurt or lay you up. It's not going to make you grow a beard and sideburns. You won't have to change your hairstyle to look like a senator in ancient Rome and you won't have to tell your friends you were mugged last Saturday evening. You won't have to wear sunglasses or say you've succumbed to a major bout of food-poisoning. And, best of all, you won't have to tap into your 401(k) program. Facebuilder is your other avenue here. Remember when Robert Frost talked about the fork in the road in his book *The Road Not Taken*? You do have a choice here. Take the Facebuilder path. It's the road to a natural, well-toned sculpted face that will last you a lifetime.

Assessing your face

It's very important that you become familiar with your face before you start the Facebuilder program. You need to be just as aware of your face's pleasing features as of any flaws you may feel you have. It's going to be important to understand the reasons for your facial flaws. This knowledge will be indispensable as you work toward correcting the flaws. Becoming familiar with your face now will help you spot the progress you make.

At this stage it's also necessary to understand how important a factor your lifestyle plays in facial appearance. What you eat and drink, how much sleep you average, the exercises you do to keep fit and your exposure to the elements all have a major impact on how you feel and, more importantly, on how you look. These are all factors that cannot be neglected. Read Chapter 6 for more information.

Now, take several photographs of your face, both front and profile, to honestly assess your face. Don't smile in either photo. After exercising your face for several weeks, take another couple of photographs posing in the same manner. Remember that our minds can play tricks and we can't always trust ourselves to be objective. The camera is not biased, however. It's not going to give any false illusions. Keep in mind that it's important to know how you *really* look, not how you *think* you really look. Have you ever looked at a candid picture of yourself, in a crowd or whatever, and uttered, "I don't think I look like that"? I'm sure you have. Well, guess what? That *is* how you really look. Remember, the camera doesn't lie.

Some good news here. You're going to see a difference in your "before" and "after" photos if you've been doing the exercises faithfully. Here's some better news. Your face will continue to make positive changes as long as you keep up the exercise program. When you make up your mind to really stick with the Facebuilder program, your face will reap huge dividends. Commit to the exercises and they will commit to you. But as I like to say to my clients, "Do it big or stay in bed."

Lines and wrinkles

Let's face it. Every face has lines. Even brand-new babies have lines and wrinkles. Some people like to say that face lines *add* character. I say that face lines *add age* and make you look like an *old* character. Who needs that look? Mark Twain once said, "Today's wrinkles are yesterday's smiles." I would paraphrase Mr. Twain by saying that yesterday's smiles *don't have* to be today's wrinkles. Not with Facebuilder on your side. And, let's not forget that there are different types of facial lines. Not all wrinkles are lines and vice versa. It's a fact. By having a good understanding of how these lines differ, you will be able to objectively study and know your face. I identify five different categories of lines:

Built-in lines These are lines formed over the years by our habitual expressions and they give the face an individual identity. Many of these lines are hereditary. Some people question things so frequently that they form what I call the "question mark" lines between the brows. Other people squint habitually, which will give you crow's feet faster than you can say it. And then there are those "tension" lines, brought on by the daily stress of everyday living.

Sleep lines These are the lines I like to refer to as the "night-time enemy." Face muscles are working, even as you are sleeping, insidiously and relentlessly creating skin lines and wrinkles without you even knowing it. And, if you are one of those people who bury your face in your pillow each night, you'll eventually look like Methuselah, who was 969 years old when he checked out. Or maybe Rip Van Winkle. Do you remember Rip's face? I call him Rip Van Wrinkle—the man who took that twenty-year "power nap." You can bet he had his face so buried in his pillow that you couldn't tell where his face stopped and the pillow started. In a nutshell, don't sleep with your face in the pillow. Better yet, don't sleep with a pillow at all.

Lines due to collapsed muscles The stomach isn't the only part of the body to sag as the body ages. The facial muscles begin to collapse as well if they are not properly exercised. This will cause many new lines to appear in the skin as we age.

Scar lines These lines are the result of injury, infection or other disorders of the skin. By toning the facial muscles, Facebuilder can help to restore the natural elasticity of the skin, improve the circulation to the face and create a smoother appearance facially.

Sun lines If you've spent years in the sun (as I did), you're going to have fine lines from all that sunbathing when you were younger. It's a shame that a tan looks so macho and healthy. In reality, sunbathing is actually very unhealthy and harmful; it can cause cancer not to mention a range of other disorders. The problem of photoaging (skin damage due to exposure to the sun) absolutely cannot be overstated. The medical community long ago publicized the negative effects the sun has on the skin. Dr. Wilma Bergfield, a past president of the American Academy of Dermatology, is quoted as saying that "our skin would remain smooth and firm for years longer if we exercised more effective sun protection." As if any more proof were needed, the *Jour-*

nal of the National Cancer Institute found that people who used tanning devices were one and a half to two times more likely to have common kinds of skin cancer than people who did not use tanning devices. That's a fact and we all have to *face it.*

Factors affecting the skin

If you consume a lot of alcohol and caffeinated drinks, such as coffee, tea and cola, and rarely drink water to flush out your system, you could have a whole host of skin problems. Mild dehydration contributes to bags under the eyes, sallow skin, blemishes, acne and numerous other skin problems. Water is an indispensable element to our well-being and we should drink at least eight glasses every day of our lives. I know W. C. Fields was once quoted as saying that he never drank water because of the disgusting things fish did in it, but let's never forget that our bodies are 70 percent water and drinking water is an excellent way to keep the skin clear and smooth. Let's also never forget that W. C. Fields consumed copious amounts of another type of beverage to get his complexion to look the way it did. His body was probably 70 percent alcohol.

While your energy levels, personality and emotional make-up influence your facial appearance, you also need to remember that heredity still plays a major role in facial features and bone structure. As you study your face, you will probably notice some things you've inherited from your ancestors and the older we get, the more pronounced these features become. After a while we start to resemble our mothers and fathers. Physical traits can definitely be passed down from generation to generation. Did your father furrow his brows when he was under pressure? Did your mother purse her lips when things were not going smoothly? Did someone in your family grimace, frown or distort his or her face when the stress thermometer was heading south? If any of these things seem familiar, relax. Don't stress. If you don't want to resemble those individuals, you have the ability to re-route or at least seriously delay Father Time's inexorable journey across your face. Doing Facebuilder can help to counteract these inherited traits. Just keep working on it and be conscious of the traits in the first place.

Continue to review your "before" photograph as you progress. Make up your mind as to what you feel are your positive and negative attributes. Which features do you wish to improve? Which features do you want to minimize? Be totally objective here. Look at that face in the photograph and focus on the changes you want to make. Write them down. Do your Facebuilder exercises regularly and see how dramatically you can change those facial areas.

Before and after—the evidence

Take a look at the truly amazing results achieved by Matthew Sanchez. His "before" picture was taken when he was twenty-eight. His face has an overall puffy appearance. His eyes appear tired and he was being told he looked tired by his associates. Matt says, "My face looks fatigued." His face also exhibits an overall lack of muscle tone and he has a dull complexion. His face lacks definition and his jawline was soft. Matt's "after"

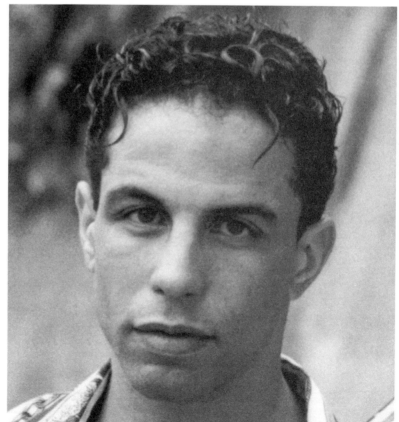

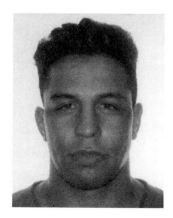

picture was snapped a year later. His face now shows strong definition and good overall muscle tone. His eyes have opened up and his upper and lower eyelids have lifted. Matt's jawline is strong, his complexion has a healthy appearance and his face has much more definition. You can see how his cheeks have developed. To quote Matt, "I presently work out my face for about seven minutes twice a day. I do my facial exercises when I wake up, when I drive and I repeat the procedure before I go to sleep. I enjoy the exercises and I look forward to doing them. These exercises have endowed me with the knowledge that I have the ability to change my facial features. I personally have that power. No surgeons, no pills, nothing except my desire for improvement." Matt went from looking average to looking like a magazine cover model. All of this was accomplished naturally.

Now have a look at the following "before" and "after" pictures of three fellows who did the Facebuilder exercises for twenty-one days. Imagine what the changes would be after two or three months? Imagine after a year or two?

The five signs of aging

Here is a summary of the five main signs of facial aging:

1. Low eyebrows When the muscle tone around the eyes weakens, the area under the eyebrows begin to look low and heavy. This is especially true when viewed from the profile. By doing the Eyebrow Lift (see p. 56), you will be able to strengthen the eyebrow and scalp muscles so that the brow arch is lifted naturally. You'll also strengthen the tiny, vital muscles in the eyelids, which will keep the eyelids lifted, resulting in the eye area looking smooth and youthful.

2. Drooping eyelids Let's face it, guys. Virtually all men eventually get drooping eyelids. Some sooner than others, but virtually no one escapes this facial scourge completely. That's why the eyelift is the most popular plastic surgery procedure being performed on men today. The number one hit on the plastic surgery hit parade.

Drooping or heavy eyelids can be a family trait or the cruel results of aging. Most probably it's a combination of both. The Eye Toner exercise (see p. 52) will strengthen the upper eyelids so that the muscles become stronger and the eyes open up, making them appear larger and more youthful. More vibrant, open eyes will make you look much more alert and "with it." A real plus. It will really give you the edge in business.

3. Lack of facial definition Here we have what I like to refer to as the GAG effect. GAG is an acronym for Genetics, Age and Gravity. It's also what you probably do when you peruse the effects these things have on your face over the long-

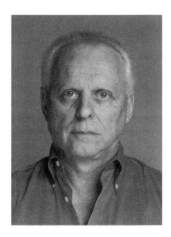

First day M.G., age sixty-one. M.G.'s face exhibits a stressed, tired appearance and an overall lack of facial tone. His jawline lacks definition. His eyes look tired.

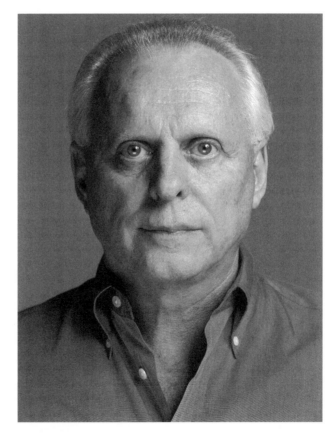

Twenty-first day M.G.'s face has taken on a much more toned appearance. His face seems more rested and he looks more youthful. His jawline is more defined and his eyes exhibit a more open, alert appearance.

term. Not a pretty picture, is it? No Kodak moment, that's for sure. Unfortunately, the three elements that make up GAG are tireless nuisances, which are constantly at work making you look worse than you deserve to appear. Your face begins to lose its definition. Your cheeks start to look lower and flatter on your face. Your face takes on that "I've been up for days and I need some sleep" appearance. In a word, you're not looking so hot. The Face Toner exercise (see p. 58) can build and beef up your facial muscles so that the cheeks appear higher and more defined on your face. After a few days of doing this exercise, you'll begin to feel

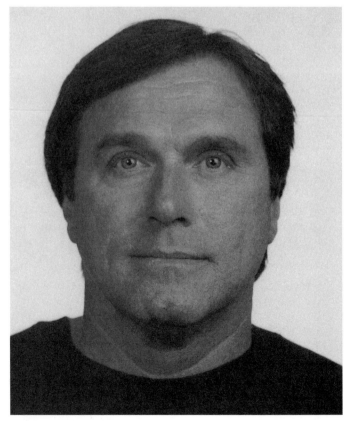

First day Steve, age forty-two. Steve's face shows heavy hooding around the upper eyelid area and he exhibits an overall lack of facial definition. His jawline is slack.

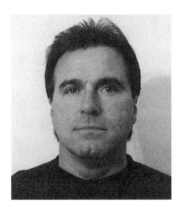

Twenty-first day Steve's eyes are much more open and youthful looking. His face has more definition and it exhibits good overall muscle tone. His jawline looks strong and defined. Steve was so impressed with his facial improvements that he is now a licensed Facebuilder instructor in the Boston area.

your cheek muscles move as they are developing. Men tell me it's like finally being able to feel a bicep work after doing curls for a while when they first start to lift weights. They tell me that they know they are making headway when they can feel the cheek muscles move. No more GAGing when you look in the mirror after a few weeks of Facebuilder.

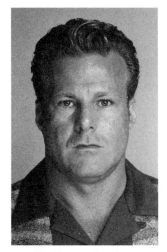

First day Scott, age thirty-four. Scott has oily skin which creates an overall dull, saggy- looking appearance. His face lacks definition and his jawline is soft. He has a slight double chin. His eyes look tired and he has a slight frown line on his forehead.

Twenty-first day Scott's skin has tightened with increased circulation and blood flow to the facial area. His face is more defined and his jawline looks stronger. His double chin has virtually disappeared. His eyes have a more open, youthful appearance. The frown line in his forehead has smoothed out and is virtually invisible now.

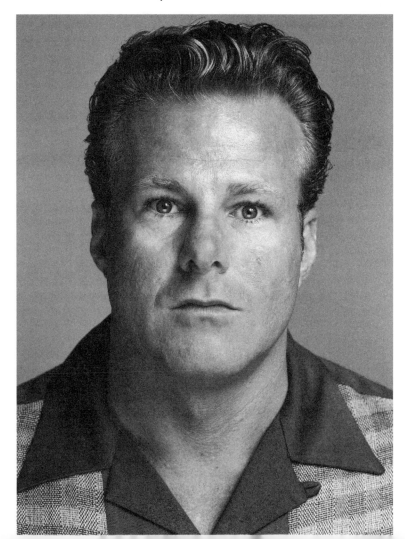

4. Nose faults Remember Pinocchio? He was a little boy puppet who magically came to life, but whenever he told a lie, his nose would start to grow. As we get older, we don't have to lie to get our noses to do this. It just happens naturally. As cheek muscles slacken and start to sag, a hollow area starts to develop around the sides of your nose. While gravity pulls the nose down, the muscles around the mouth gradually begin to lose their shape and their tone. This nature-induced double whammy contributes to sagging and gives you the appearance of having just found out you have a visitor from the IRS. To keep yourself from being mistaken for Pinocchio, you need to develop the tiny nasal muscle located under each nostril. By doing the Nose Toner exercise (see p. 60) daily, you'll improve the appearance of the nose as well as of the upper lip. This exercise really works well. So well that many politicians worldwide have been using it for years.

5. Sagging jawline and/or double chin We all know that a strong, defined jawline gives a man a sense of confidence and assurance. Heredity plays a vital part in the shape and tone of the jawline and chin, as I've mentioned before. By the age of thirty or so, many men find that their jawline and chin are starting to sag, losing definition and tone. The result is a weak, aged appearance. You can dramatically improve the firmness and tone of the jawline area by doing the Jaw Toner and the Double Chin Toner (see p. 66 and 72).

Anthony Powell once said that growing old was being increasingly penalized for a crime you didn't commit. He was right. But while aging *is* a fact of life, Facebuilder is going to make sure you're not penalized for growing older. Now that you've had a chance to study your "before" photographs and have had a chance to reflect on the good and bad points of your facial features, it's time to go for it. You have the "before" pictures. Let's start the journey to those "after" pictures, which you'll want to show everyone. Seeing is believing, and the "after" pictures are going to make believers out of anyone who stays with the program.

4

Your facial muscles

Where they are, what they're called, how they work

Most men have a general understanding of the muscles of the body and how they work. They also understand that certain exercise programs will keep these muscles strong and toned. Millions of health- and age-conscious men have already started an exercise program. They are pec-pumping, stepping, running on treadmills, jogging, ab-crunching, spinning—you name it. They know that these exercises will quickly develop a better-looking body. Most men, however, have virtually no understanding of their facial muscles, what they are called or how they work. So, for all of you who took anatomy classes at college because you needed the sleep, here's a refresher course on what you missed.

The human face has fifty-seven muscles which work together to support and maintain the facial features. With every facial movement you make, from furrowing your brow, laughing at a joke or even powering down a doughnut before anyone sees you (known as a "power pop"), your facial muscles are working in synergy to perform myriad functions, creating the expressions we all see each day.

Possessing a working knowledge of the facial muscles and being able to picture their location and capabilities will assist you in creating the mind-muscle connection that is so important to successful facial development. This is the fundamental foundation of the Facebuilder program. You will be consciously using your mind to exercise your facial muscles and your exercise program will be successful because it is built on rock-hard Facebuilder experience.

When you begin to learn the Facebuilder exercises, you'll be able to feel your muscles move and flex, just as you would if you were exercising the biceps, calf muscles or other muscles of the body. Facial muscles resemble a patchwork quilt lying just beneath the surface of the skin, connected by bundles of fibers. I consider these muscles magical because of the artistic feats they perform. Working with their connective fibers, these muscles give our faces life, animation and all the expressions that make each of us so unique. Without these acrobatic muscles, our faces would be mask-like, expressionless and, frankly, quite boring.

Facebuilder hones all the muscles of the face, neck and scalp. The muscles are interconnected, so they are all working together. When you begin your Facebuilder regime, it's vitally important that you do the exercises in the order in which they are given in this book. When you do an exercise, you are working a particular group of muscles in the face. When you move on to the next exercise, the first group of muscles begins recuperating and rebuilding. Being aware of the facial muscles and using your visualization powers to expand the muscle's activities (seeing it get larger or feeling it move) are all part of the Facebuilder concept of mind-muscle connection. You'll need to focus and concentrate to remain in this state of mind. If you do this, you'll start to see some amazing changes in your face in a short period of time. The longer you continue to do the exercises, the better the mind-muscle connection will be and the more effective the exercises will become. Take a few minutes to study the muscle groups and locate them on the illustration on page 41. Possessing a rudimentary working knowledge of your facial muscles, their location and what they do will definitely help you in bringing your best face forward.

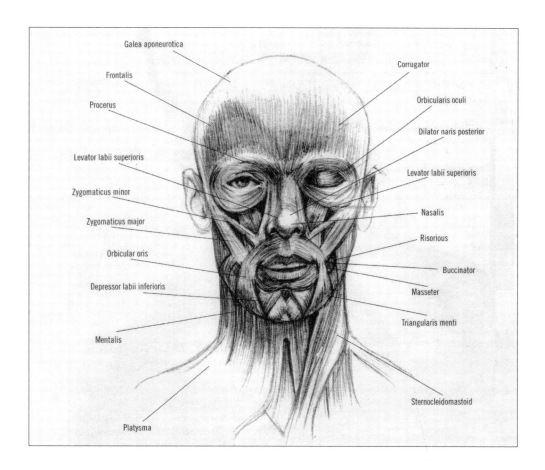

Galea aponeurotica

Frontalis

Procerus

Levator labii superioris

Zygomaticus minor

Zygomaticus major

Orbicular oris

Depressor labii inferioris

Mentalis

Platysma

Corrugator

Orbicularis oculi

Dilator naris posterior

Levator labii superioris

Nasalis

Risorious

Buccinator

Masseter

Triangularis menti

Sternocleidomastoid

Muscles of the scalp

The skin of the scalp is the thickest skin on the human body (which might account for the term hardheaded).

■ Beneath the skin are a number of scalp muscles, including the *epicranius*, which is divided into different areas.

■ The *frontalis* is one part of the *epicranius*. It is a thin muscle located over the forehead. It raises the eyebrows and the skin over the root of the nose. It also simultaneously draws the scalp forward, throwing the skin of the forehead into transverse wrinkles. In layman's language, a frown. The Eyebrow Lift strengthens the *frontalis*, lifting and toning it, which keeps forehead wrinkles from forming.

■ The *occipitalis* measures about an inch and a half long and lies at the back of the head. It is also part of the *epicranius*. This muscle draws the scalp backward. Again, the Eyebrow Lift enhances this muscle, with the same results it achieves with the *frontalis*. The entire scalp may be moved forward and backward by the activity of these two muscles.

■ The *galea aponeurotica* is a broad, flat tendon that covers the upper part of the cranium, joining the *frontalis* and *occipitalis* muscles. It also benefits from the Eyebrow Lift.

Are we having fun yet?

Muscles of the mouth

■ The *orbicularis oris* completely encircles the mouth. It consists of numerous strata of muscular fibers, which travel in different directions and connect with fibers in the upper and lower lips, cheeks, nose and the surrounding areas. This muscle is responsible for the closure of the lips. The Mouth Toner is a great exercise for firming and toning this muscle and, consequently, the lips.

■ The *buccinator* is a thin, quadrilateral structure occupying the space between the maxilla and the mandible (upper and lower jawbones) at each side of the face. This muscle assists in the act of sucking. The Face Toner and Facelift work wonders on this muscle, helping to tone and strengthen it.

■ The *mentalis* is a tiny muscle in the front of the chin. It raises the chin and makes the lower lip protrude (a pout) and it also wrinkles the skin of the chin. The Mouth Toner will firm up this muscle.

■ Next up is the *quadratus labii superioris*. This is a broad sheet of muscle, which lies around the upper lip and is connected to the cheek muscle. Its function is to raise the lip (a snarl). The Mouth Toner and the Face Toner are just the ticket for exercising this muscle.

■ The *quadratus labii inferioris* is a small, quadrilateral muscle which draws down the lower lip (kind of a mini pout). The Mouth Toner will help keep this muscle firm and toned.

■ Last but not least, we have the *caninus*. This is the sneer muscle. This little guy raises the upper lip to form a sneer. Keeping this muscle in shape is a job for the Mouth Toner.

Muscles of the nose

It's important to understand that the muscles of the nose work closely together. The Nose Toner benefits all of these muscles in different ways.

■ First we have the *procerus*. This pyramidal muscle crosses the bridge of the nose. Its function is to pull down the middle of the eyebrows and it produces transverse wrinkles over the bridge of the nose. Not a pretty picture, is it? Well, there's good news here—the Nose Toner. This exercise will help to counteract the effects the *procerus* produces.

■ The *nasalis* is a muscle that begins at the bridge of the nose and extends upward over the bridge of the nose, compressing the nostrils. The Nose Toner helps here, too.

■ Next we have the *depressor septi*. This muscle extends across the base of the nose and closes the nasal openings by pulling down the septum (the cartilage partition between the nostrils). Practicing the Nose Toner will help to tone the muscle and keep the nose from growing longer and/or wider.

■ The *dilatator naris posterior* is next on the list. It lies near the margin of the nostril and it acts to increase the size of the nasal opening, allowing more air into the lungs.

■ Finally we have the *dilatator naris anterior*. This is a thin and delicate muscle, which lies directly above the middle of each nostril. This muscle also opens the nostrils, causing them to flare.

Muscles of mastication

These are the muscles used in the opening and closing of the jaws, for example in chewing or yawning. Many of you fellows hold the tensions of the day in your jaw area. Knowing the location of these muscles and how to work them can help you alleviate these tensions with the added benefit of helping to build up the muscle tone in your face. The Jaw Toner is the *exercise de jour* here. It exercises all of the above muscles and helps keep them toned, defined and firm. No slack jaw here.

■ The *masseter* and the *temporalis* work in conjunction with each other to close the teeth with force, as when chewing food or gum. Unfortunately, they also collaborate to grind your teeth in your sleep.

■ Next up we have the *pterygoideus externus*. This short, thick muscle is somewhat cone-shaped. It assists in opening the mouth and rotating the jaw.

■ The *pterygoideus internus* is another thick, quadrilateral muscle. It contributes to the crushing, grinding action of the jaw.

Muscles of the eye

■ The *orbicularis oculi* is a powerful muscle that surrounds the orbit of the eye. It acts involuntarily to close the eyelids gently, as when you sleep or blink. When the entire muscle is brought into action, the skin moves in folds, which radiate from the outer corners of the eyelids. These folds form those infamous crow's feet. The Facebuilder exercise called the Eye Toner will teach you how to exercise this muscle without creating folds in the skin. Correct finger placement is the key to success in this exercise.

■ The *levator palpebra superioris* is a thin muscle in the upper eyelid. It maintains the firmness of the upper eyelid and keeps it from drooping. The Eye Toner will help to keep this muscle toned and taut and will help you to maintain that youthful, open-eyed look.

■ There is also the *epicranius*. This muscle raises the eyebrows. Exercising the *epicranius* increases oxygen and blood circulation throughout the forehead and eye areas.

Regular exercise of this muscle can soften your brows and give you a more relaxed appearance.

"The eyes are the windows to the world." That's how Dr. Gerald Walman, Medical Director at ImageCare Laser Centers in Scottsdale, Arizona, so poignantly puts it. He correctly points out that the eyes are probably the most important areas of the face because when people first meet they are drawn to each other's eyes. Eye contact is the first thing any successful person needs to develop if they are going to succeed in the business world. Any improvements that can be made in the rejuvenation of the eyelid area has got to be the number one most effective way to improve our image.

Dr. Walman once told me that he was impressed at the variations in the muscle tone that could be observed with the passage of time and how this muscle tone directly relates to the aesthetics of the facial area. He went on to state that individuals over forty usually exhibit an increased loosening and laxity of the eyelid tissues, generally caused by loss of elasticity in the underlying tissues, which are supported by the *orbicularis oculi* muscle. This loss of elasticity leads to bulging of the fat pads within the orbit surrounding the eyes, leading to bags under the eyes. This loss of muscle tone also contributes to wrinkles and crow's feet. Dr. Walman should know. He has over twenty-two years of experience in ophthalmology and ocular-plastic surgery. He also told me that regular facial exercises which work the *orbicularis oculi* muscle and other facial muscles surrounding the eye area *will* increase tone and thus decrease the severity of wrinkles, crow's feet and other problems that afflict the delicate skin surrounding the eye. What can I say to improve on that? The doctor knows best.

Muscles of the neck

■ The *platysma* is a broad thin plane of muscular fibers lying under the skin on each side of the neck. This is a powerful muscle and it produces oblique wrinkles in the neck and depresses the lower jaw. The Jaw Toner and Double Chin Toner are excellent exercises for toning and honing this muscle so that the skin smoothes out over the neck area.

■ As well as being a very long word, the *sternocleidomastoid* is the muscle that rotates the head and turns it to either side. This is a fairly large muscle, which is thick, broad and very powerful. The Jaw Toner and Double Chin Toner exercises work very well on this muscle, keeping it toned and strong.

■ We also have the *trapezius*. This muscle is located at the back of the neck and shoulders. It turns the head from side to side and works in tandem with the *sternocleidomastoid*. (There's that word again.) The Jaw Toner and Double Chin Toner exercises work on this muscle as well, with equally positive results.

Muscles of the ear

There are three small muscles, which lie right under the skin surrounding the ear. These muscles have very little effect on facial appearance, but they are interconnected to other muscles that *do* have a *big* effect on the overall toning and honing of the face through Facebuilder. It is very important to learn how to make these little muscles move so as to achieve optimum results in strengthening and defining your scalp and facial muscles. When you are doing exercises designed to firm up your jawline, for instance, concentrate on flexing your ears. This will help you focus on the jaw muscle groups and will enhance the exercise. Additionally, when you are doing exercises that lift and tone the upper eye and eyebrow area, flexing the ears will help ease frown lines around the eyes.

■ The *anterior auricularis* is the smallest ear muscle. Thin and fan-shaped, it assists in drawing the ears forwards. When you are doing the scooping movement in the Jaw Toner exercise, remember to concentrate on flexing the ears.

■ The *superior auricularis* is the largest of the ear muscles. Its function is to raise the ears. While this movement may seem almost nonexistent, when you are doing the Facelift exercise, concentrate on this muscle. You should visualize your ears lifting as you visualize the sides of your face moving up. Don't be discouraged if you don't see or feel it move. It is the visualization of the muscle movement that assists you in exercising the surrounding muscles.

■ The *posterior auricularis* draws the ears backward. When you are doing the Face Strengthening exercise, imagine pushing your ears backward as you mentally expand the sides of your face. This will help you to visualize the sides of your face widening. It's this action that actually makes your face wider and fills in the gaunt, drawn area of the lower face.

Ready to begin

Now we've introduced the major players in the face. I know it sounds like we've just taken a trip through *Jurassic Park*, with all those muscle names that sound like names of different dinosaurs. Well, they're only dinosaurs if you don't exercise them, guys. It's time to put all those muscles with funny names to work for you, not against you. You're ready to introduce your face to Facebuilder, which is about to change the way you look at yourself and the way others look at you. Seeing is believing. Facebuilder is going to be your ticket for a fantastic journey—a journey that ends with a more dynamic, younger-looking you. So hop onboard, guys. This is an e-ticket ride you're not going to want to miss.

5

Let's go for it

Eleven face-strengthening exercises

Facebuilder teaches you skills that are gradually perfected through daily practice. Consistency is the important concept here. These exercises will become second nature in a matter of weeks and you will start to see a firmer jawline, a rapidly receding double chin and much more youthful-looking eyes.

Facebuilder has a tremendous advantage over many other exercise programs in that it is flexible, safe, easy, and can be done anywhere, any time. You don't need anything you weren't born with to perform these exercises. For example, you can do the Mouth Toner exercise while you work on the computer. While talking on the phone, you can practice the Nose Toner. At work, if you catch yourself drifting off mentally, you can do two sets of the Eye Toner exercise to increase the circulation around your eyes. This will boost your concentration big time. As you master these exercises, you will find yourself automatically doing them because they make your face feel pumped and energized. They are a kind of a mini-workout for the face and provide that same nice afterglow you get after doing some strength training exercises in the gym.

As with anything important in your life, you need to schedule Facebuilder into your daily routine from the very start. A good way to begin your day is to do each Facebuilder exercise once, as soon as you wake up. The whole routine will only take up about ten minutes of your morning. You can even do them while lying in bed. They're a great wake-up call. These exercises will energize you and help to reduce the puffiness around the eyes and face. You'll notice that your face will look more toned as you shave, giving you a cool, clean-cut appearance. What's wrong with that? In the evening, I suggest you do each exercise again. This way you'll get in your two sessions daily and your face will be relaxed and ready for some good sack time.

If you're like most people I know, you're living life in the fast lane. Time is important and no one I know has enough of it. It's important that you make time to do constructive things for yourself, however. That's why I have developed a sequence of exercises that can be done while you are driving your car.

To obtain the noticeable results you want, you'll need to do the exercises twice daily for three to four weeks, while you are in the learning stage. Most of my clients find that after investing a few months of disciplined workouts, they've knocked from five to ten years off their appearance. People *will* notice and they *will* comment on the changes they observe. They'll say things to you like, "Hey, have you had a new hair cut?" "Did you lose some weight?" "Have you started exercising?" "You look different." You won't get tired of hearing those comments, I can assure you, especially when the ladies start saying it. Once you have achieved the initial benefits you started out to obtain, you'll probably want to move on to a maintenance program in which you do the exercises as your face needs them. Make Facebuilder your unseen helper—your secret weapon in fending off the aging process.

Read through all the exercise directions several times before initiating the exercises. Just as you focus on a certain group of muscles while exercising in the gym, you will want to focus on the facial muscles you are exercising in the same way. Keep in mind that it takes longer to build body muscles because they are bigger than facial muscles. Your face is going to react much more quickly to these Facebuilder exercises so the results will be noticeable in a short period of time. It's going to be a quick trip to a younger appearance. When you start to see the positive results you're going to achieve, you'll know you're right around the corner from looking better than ever.

Five tips to remember

1. Basic position Before you do each exercise, to prepare yourself, suck in your stomach, tighten your bottom and hold. This position anchors you so that you can focus on the individual facial muscles you are exercising. *Now, remember:* Each time you see the words "Assume the basic position" as you read through these exercises, I want you to assume the posture defined above. Doing the exercises in this position will ensure you get the best results.

2. Lactic acid burn Concentrate and focus on the muscle group you are working until you feel a tight, achy feeling. The exertion creates a build-up of lactic acid in the muscle and the burning sensation is a sign that the muscle is being worked to its maximum capacity. Jimmy Conners came up with the phrase "No pain. No gain." Toni Anderson later paraphrased it to "No pain. No pain." That's funny, but we all know that Jimmy is right if we want to develop our facial muscles. So let's go for the lactic acid burn, guys.

3. Pulsing In facial exercising you use your fingertips as counterweights. They provide the resistance necessary for the muscle to work harder and grow stronger so that you achieve results as quickly as possible. I have a term I call "pulsing." It means moving your fingers quickly up and down your face at the muscle points to intensify the lactic acid burn. Don't forget this term. You'll need to remember it always. It works.

4. Focus When you do the exercises, stay focused and feel the energy coursing through your muscles as they work. Picture the muscles you are exercising lifting and starting to move up your face. When you read through the following exercises, you will see that I often say, "Follow the energy in your face." My concept of energy flow is based on the traditional Chinese medicinal theory that energy moves in pathways throughout the body. I know from experience that feeling and focusing on the energy flow helps people to master the exercise techniques more quickly. If you visualize the energy flowing around your body your facial muscles will develop more quickly than if you do not.

5. Blow away Press your lips together and blow between them, making sure that you vibrate the lips. You'll be doing this routine after each exercise to relax your facial muscles and "blow away" the lactic-acid burning ache.

Exercise 1

Eye Toner

Benefits

The Eye Toner exercises the *orbicularis oculi*, the muscle that surrounds the entire eye. One of the most important muscles in the body, this muscle opens and closes the eye. The Eye Toner pumps blood into the whole eye area and strengthens the upper and lower eyelids. It works to reduce under-eye puffiness, lift under-eye hollows and, in effect, enlarge the eye socket, giving you a more wide-awake, bright-eyed look. How is that possible? Here are the facts: As we age, the upper eyelid muscles lose their tone and sag down in the eye socket, invading that area and making it appear

Method

1. Perform this exercise lying down or in a sitting position. Assume the basic position (see p. 50). Place your index fingers between your brows, then wrap your thumbs lightly around the outer eye corners, on top of your crow's feet (if you have them). Look up toward the top of your head. Make a strong squint upward with the lower eyelid.

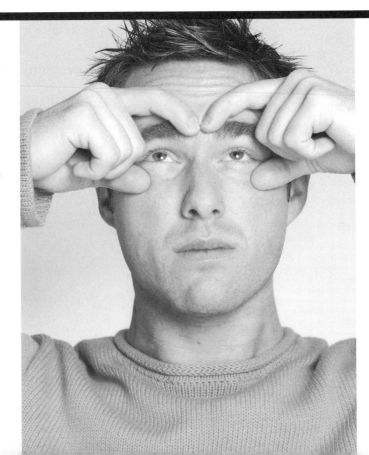

smaller. By toning and lifting the upper and lower eyelids, the eye socket becomes more defined and appears larger.

Tip: Perform the Eye Toner twice a day. If you have deep hollows or severe under-eye puffiness, repeat the exercise three times daily. You should apply slight pressure with your index fingers, pulling up between the brows. This action will prevent your eyebrows furrowing or wrinkling. Keep your thumbs at your outer-eye corners, applying light pressure only, so as not to create creases in your skin.

2. Hold the squint and squeeze your eyes tightly shut, keeping your buttocks clenched tightly, and count to forty. It's *very important* to keep your eyes closed tightly and your bottom tightened as you count.

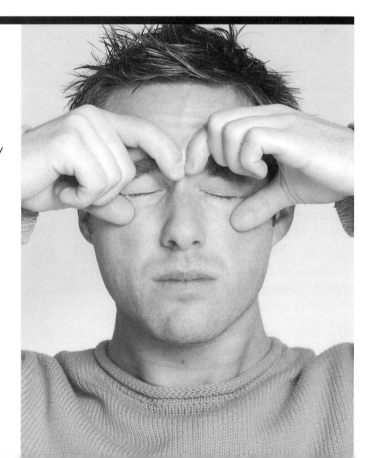

Exercise 2

Lower Eyelid Lift

Benefits This exercise also strengthens the *orbicularis oculi* muscle. It is useful for firming the lower eyelids, diminishing the hollows under the eyes and reducing under-eye puffiness.

Method

1. You can do this exercise either sitting or lying down. I alternate positions to work the muscle differently. Assume the basic position (see p. 50). Place your index fingers at your outer-eye corners and your middle fingers at your inner-eye corners and apply light pressure. Look up towards the top of your head. Make a strong squint upward with your lower eyelids. Squint up and release five times, keeping your upper eyelids wide open.

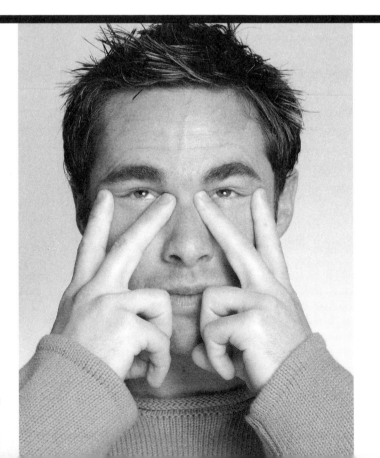

Tip: Perform the Lower Eyelid Lift twice a day. If you have extensive eye puffiness, repeat this exercise three times a day. As you do the exercise remember to maintain a slight pressure with your fingers at the outer- and inner-eye corners to keep the skin from creasing.

2. Hold this squint and think *up*, maintaining a strong squint with your lower eyelids. Remember to keep your bottom tightly clenched. Count to forty.

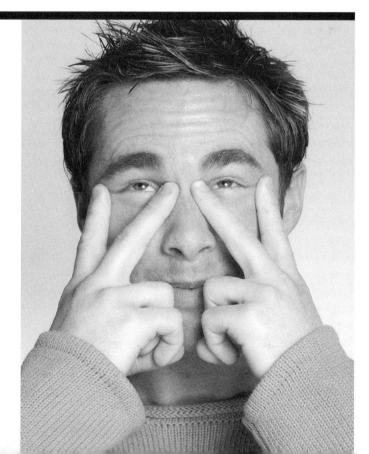

Exercise 3

Eyebrow Lift

Benefits This multipurpose exercise works the *epicranius*, which raises the eyebrows, the *frontalis*, which draws the scalp forwards, the *occipitalis*, which draws the scalp back and the *galea aponeurotica*, which joins the *frontalis* and the *occipitalis*. The Eyebrow Lift prevents or reduces the frown lines between the eyebrows and fore-

Method

1. You can do this exercise in a sitting position or lying down. I personally like to do this one lying down because I feel like I can exert more energy in this position. Assume the basic position (see p. 50). Place the index fingers of both hands in the middle of the forehead so that they are parallel to the top of each brow. Now, pull your fingers down toward your brows. Keep them held down. Look up toward the top of your head. While you are pressing down with your fingers, concentrate on pushing your eyebrows up. Push them up and release them five times.

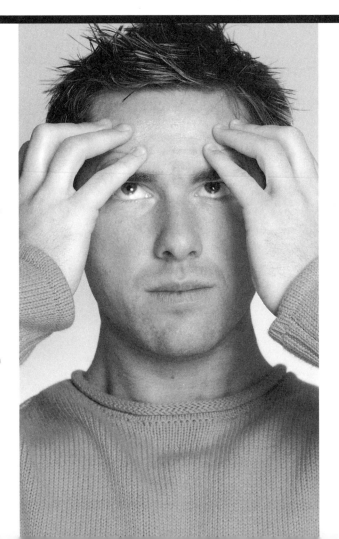

head and raises the eyebrows. It also acts to prevent or diminish the hooding effect that age and lack of muscle tone tends to cause on the upper eyelids.

Tip: Perform the Eyebrow Lift twice a day. It will help to clear your head and will make you feel much more alert. To correct a heavy or scowling brow, repeat this exercise three times a day.

2. Keeping your eyebrows in the up position, continue to keep your fingers pressed down. Do mini-eye brow pushups until you start to feel a tight band of pressure above your brows. When you feel the pressure or burn, keep your eyebrows pushed up with your fingers pushing down against them. Remember to hold your brows up. Count to thirty. Release and massage the center of your brow in a circular motion. Relaxing the muscle in this way will result in optimum development.

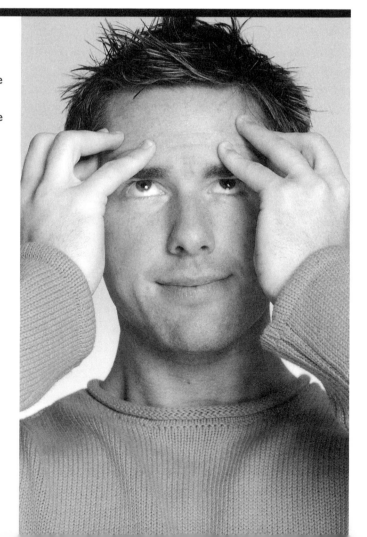

Exercise 4

Face Toner

Benefits The Face Toner harnesses the power of the mind to counteract the lengthening and flattening effects of gravity. Working the *quadratus labii superioris*, it helps to remove the stressed look from your face and increase blood circulation, giving your skin a robust appearance.

Method

1. This exercise can be done either sitting up or lying down. I prefer to do it lying down because I feel I can really push the stress out of my face in this position. Assume the basic position (see p. 50). Imagine a dot in the middle of your upper lip and a dot in the middle of your lower lip. Open your mouth, pulling those two imaginary dots apart, allowing your mouth to form an oval shape. Place your index fingers lightly on the top (apple) part of your cheeks. Smile with your mouth corners and release the corners. You should feel your cheeks move under your index fingers. Visualize the muscle under the cheek pushing up each time you smile. Repeat this movement twenty-five times. On the twenty-fifth smile, strongly pull the upper and lower lip away from each other. Imagine that your cheeks are

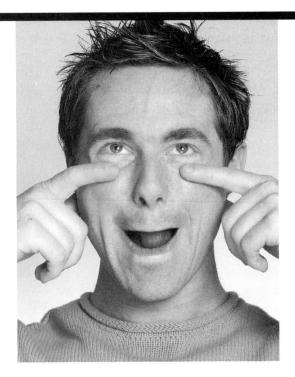

moving out from your face towards the ceiling and then exiting, like two small balloons, through the top of your scalp. Follow the energy in your face.

Tip: Do the Face Toner twice a day. If you find that you are under unusual tension or stress, do it as often as necessary. If you feel an ache in the jaw area after performing this exercise, blow out between your lips (see p. 51). This simple little act will release the lactic acid in the muscle and should give you an immediate feeling of relief.

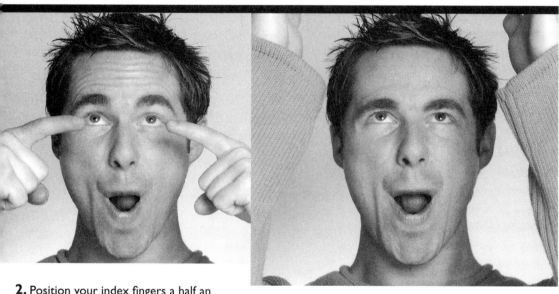

2. Position your index fingers a half an inch away from your face and then begin to move them up in front of the face, toward the scalp area. This will help you to "move" the energy of the cheeks up through the top of your head. Hold this position for a count of thirty, while looking up towards the top of your head. Move your arms above your head. Follow the energy in your face.

3. Now, if you're lying down, raise your head an inch or so, lifting your head with the front of your neck while keeping your buttocks tightened. Hold your head up, count to thirty and continue to imagine that the cheeks are moving out and up, exiting through the top of your head. Follow the energy in your face with your mind. Keep your hands outstretched above your head.

Exercise 5

Nose Toner

Benefits As I've mentioned previously, our noses continue to grow throughout our lives. The tip of the nose drops and widens with age. The good nose news here is that the Nose Toner exercise shortens and narrows the nose tip by exercising the *depressor septii* muscle. Pinocchio should have read my book. If he had, he could have kept on fibbing until the cows came home and no one would have known. Doing this exercise properly stimulates blood and oxygen flow throughout the upper lip and nose

Method

1. You can do this exercise while moving, or while sitting up or lying down. My preference is to do it while I'm on the phone. Assume the basic position (see p. 50). Push the tip of your nose up firmly with your index finger.

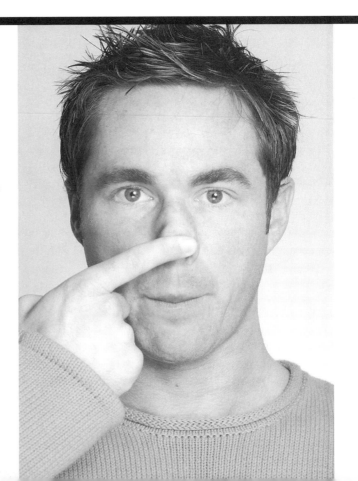

area. Many of my clients have described a tingling feeling around the nose. This is good because it shows that there is increased blood circulation to that area, which is what you want.

Tip: Do the Nose Toner once a day and if your nose is a little longer than you would like, or if it's a little too wide, carry out this exercise twice a day. Some of my clients who have had a rhinoplasty (nose job) report that doing this exercise for several weeks helps to give their nose a more naturally sculpted look.

2. Flex your nose down by pulling your upper lip down over your teeth. Hold this for a second before releasing the lip. Repeat thirty-five times. You should feel the tip of your nose push against your finger each time. Remember to keep breathing at a normal rate while you perform these repetitions.

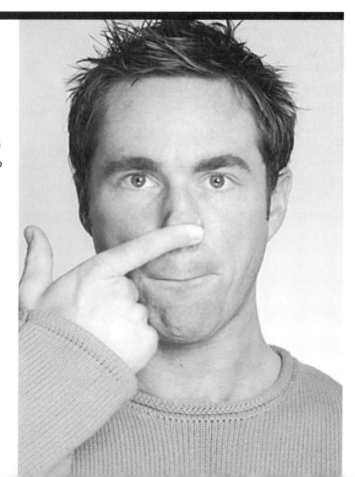

Exercise 6

Mouth Toner

Benefits By working the *orbicularis oris* muscle which encircles the mouth, the Mouth Toner strengthens the whole mouth area. One of my musician clients told me that doing this exercise strengthened his mouth, giving him the ability to play his trombone longer, which in turn lengthened his career.

Method

1. This exercise should be done sitting up. Assume the basic position (see p. 50). Press your lips together. *Do not* purse your lips and *don't* clench your teeth. Push your chin muscle up with your finger. Press the lips together and keep the tip of your nose pulled down by lowering your upper lip.

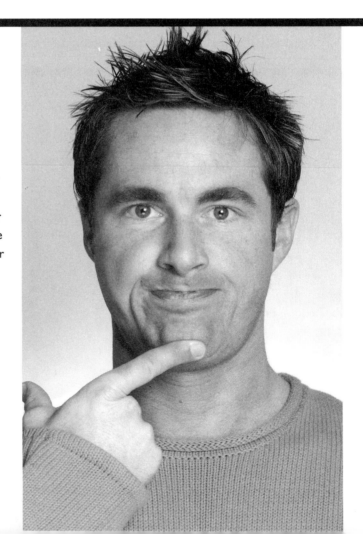

Tip: Do the Mouth Toner twice a day to strengthen your mouth. This is an excellent exercise to relieve the stress and tension many men tend to hold in the mouth area.

2. Push your face forward and your shoulders back. Keep pressing your lips together until you can feel the lactic acid burn (see p. 50) and then count to thirty before releasing. Blow out between your lips (see p. 51).

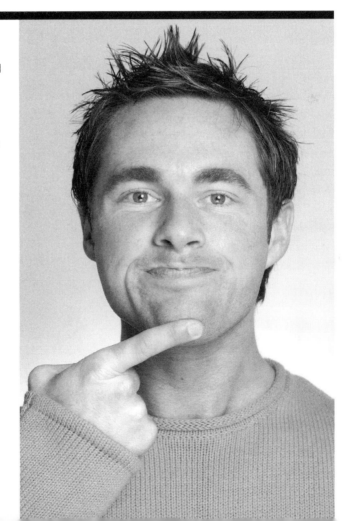

Exercise 7

Smile Line Eraser

Benefits This exercise can make a big improvement in your appearance. By building up the *dilator naris anterior* and the *dilator naris posterior* muscles, you will be able to smooth out any deep creases as well as the age lines that run from the nose to the corners of the mouth.

Method

1. This exercise is most effective when performed sitting upright. Assume the basic position (see p. 50). Imagine a dot in the center of your upper lip and a corresponding dot in the center of your lower lip. Open your mouth and pull the dots away from each other as you form a long, strong oval shape with your mouth. Remember to keep your upper lip pressing down on your teeth.

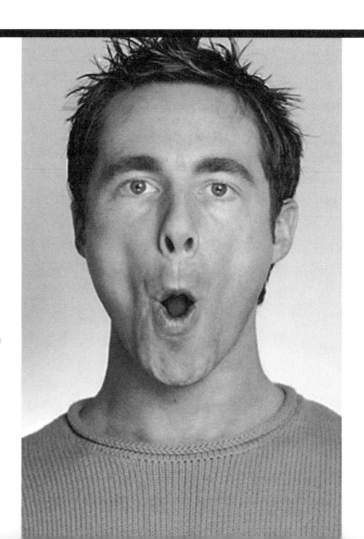

Tip: Using your powers of visualization helps to intensify the lactic acid burn and assists in developing the muscles more quickly. You should do this exercise twice a day for optimum results.

2. Visualize a line of energy moving from your mouth corners moving up to the sides of your nostrils. Use your index fingers to follow this imaginary line upward. Then visualize that energy beam moving back down the imaginary line toward your mouth corners. Repeat and use your index fingers to follow and intensify this imaginary energy. Keep this up until you feel a burn in the smile line area. When this occurs, pulse your index fingers up and down quickly to a count of thirty. Afterward blow out between your lips (see p. 51).

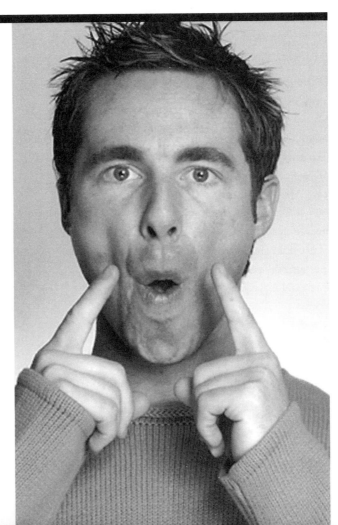

Exercise 8

Jaw Toner

Benefits This exercise benefits the *pterygoid internus* muscle in the jaw. Working this muscle will help to get rid of droopy jowls and will assist in erasing or minimizing the sagging skin along the jawline. I've been told by some of my clients that this exercise helps alleviate the painful symptoms of temporomandibular joint syndrome.

Method

1. The Jaw Toner is best done while sitting down. Assume the basic position (see p. 50). Open your mouth and roll the lower lip in securely over the bottom teeth. Pull the corners of the mouth towards the back teeth and roll them in tightly. Keep your upper lip pressed firmly against your teeth. To provide light resistance, place your index finger on your chin. Open and close your jaw in a slow scooping motion, using the corners of your mouth to open and close your jaw, not your jaw hinge. Imagine scooping up your favorite ice cream with your "scoop."

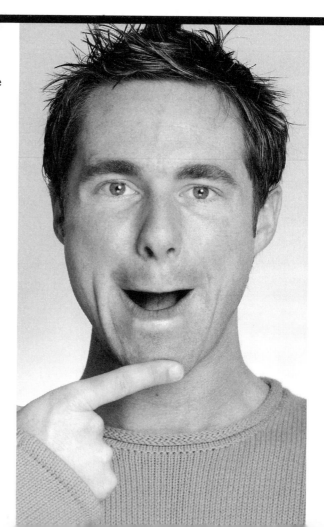

Tip: Make sure you scoop using the mouth corners, *not* the jaw hinge. Scoop slowly and deliberately. I recommend doing the Jaw Toner twice a day to help prevent a sagging jawline.

2. Pull your chin up about a half an inch each time you scoop. Scoop slowly and concentrate. Perform this motion until you get that lactic acid burning sensation in your jawline. When you feel the burn, hold your jaw still while visualizing the sides of your face lifting up. Push your face forward and your shoulders back. Concentrate on that jawline burn. Count to thirty while holding this position. Afterward blow out between your lips to relax the area (see p. 51).

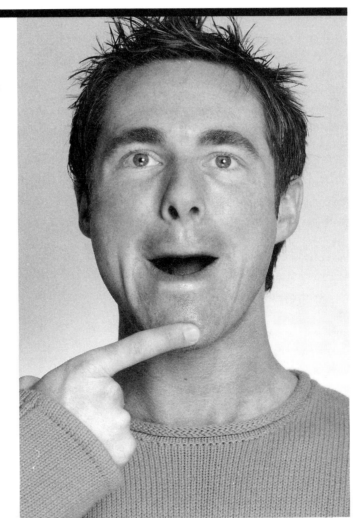

Exercise 9

Face Strengthener

Benefits This is an extremely effective exercise for long, drawn narrow faces. This one doesn't build your cheeks. It will widen and fill in that drawn look.

Method

1. This exercise can be done either sitting up or lying down. I like to do it lying down because I feel I can visualize the sides of my face expanding more easily in this position. Assume the basic position (see p. 50). Open your mouth, pull the corners of your mouth toward your back teeth and roll them in tightly. Keep your upper lip pressed down firmly against the upper teeth. Now visualize big, fat cheeks coming out of the corners of your mouth. See these fat cheeks filling in the gaunt area of your face. Position your fingertips at the corners of your mouth while making small circular motions on your face. This will mentally help you to "expand" the sides of the face. Continue making these small, circular motions.

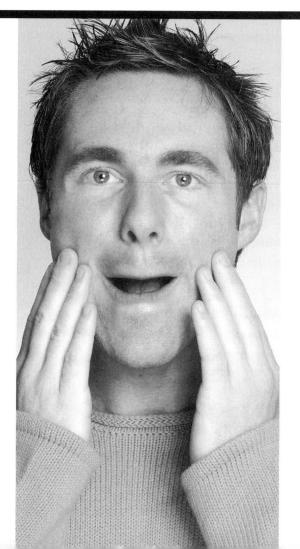

Tip: If you feel your face is wide already, you can definitely skip the Face Strengthener. Otherwise do this exercise twice a day.

2. When you begin to feel the muscle widen, slowly pull the hands away from your face while continuing the circular motions. When you begin to feel the lactic acid burn on the sides of your face, make quick circles with your fingers to intensify the energy. Continue to do this for a count of thirty. Relax and blow out between your lips (see p. 51).

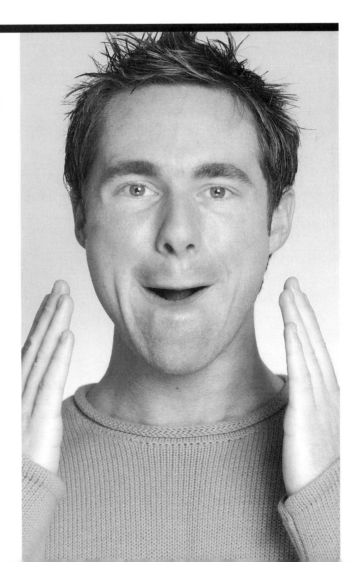

Exercise 10

Facelift

Benefits The Facelift narrows, lifts and tones your face. It exercises the *buccinator* muscle, and therefore in time will increase facial muscle tone. If your face is narrow already, you should still do this exercise once a day as it will keep the sides of your face toned.

Method

1. You can do this exercise sitting up or lying down. Personally, I like to do it lying down because I find it reverses the pull of gravity and makes it easier to do. Assume the basic position (see p. 50). Open your mouth and forcefully roll your lips over your upper and lower teeth. Pull the corners of your mouth in toward your back teeth and roll them in tightly. Place one hand on each side of your chin, then slowly move your hands up along the sides of your face, ending with the palms of your hands at eye level, as you visualize your face lifting. Use the power of your mind to help you do this exercise and visualize the sides of your face moving upward and outward, past the jawline, to the top of the head. Follow the energy in your face.

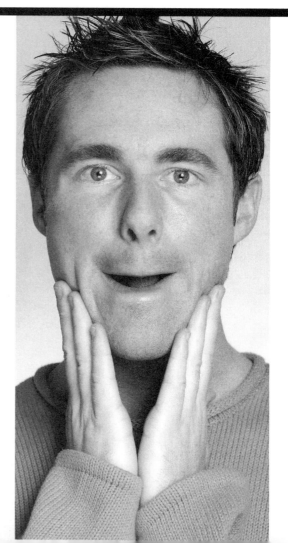

Tip: Do the facelift twice a day if you have a heavy full face. Do it once a day for general toning if your face is narrow. (If you're not sure whether your face is wide or narrow, ask a good friend.)

2. Hold the position until you feel the lactic acid burn on the sides of your face. When you achieve the burn, count to thirty. Relax and blow out between your lips (see p. 51).

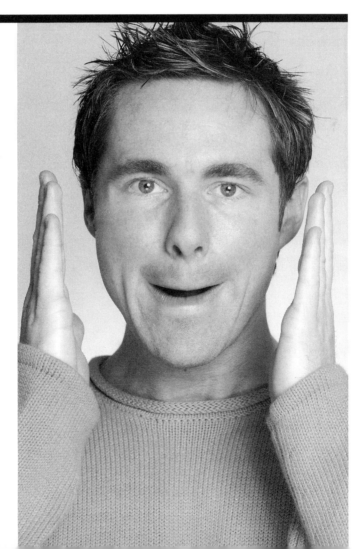

Exercise 11

Double Chin Toner

Benefits This exercise works to strengthen the *platysma* muscle. It is great for firming the chin, neck and jawline. It can greatly reduce double chins and, in some cases, make them almost invisible.

Method

1. Assume the basic position (see p. 50) and sit tall and straight with your chin held high. Close your lips and smile strongly (a smile without your teeth showing). Place both hands at the base of your throat over your collarbone and pull down slightly on the skin with a firm grip. Roll your eyes upward toward the top of your head.

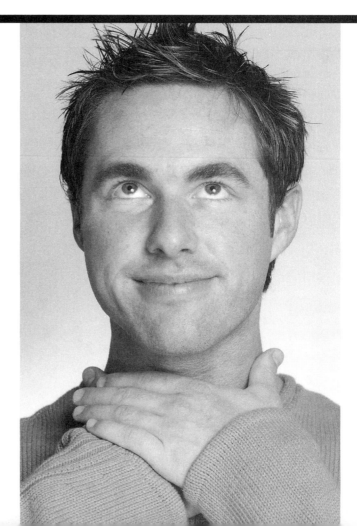

Tip: Do the Double Chin Toner twice a day and, if you feel you have a double chin problem, you can do this exercise three times a day.

2. Tilt your head back, count to three, then release. You should feel a strong pull on your chin and neck muscles. Repeat this movement thirty-five times. Then do the exercise looking over your right shoulder thirty-five times. Afterward, look over your left shoulder and do the exercise a further thirty-five times.

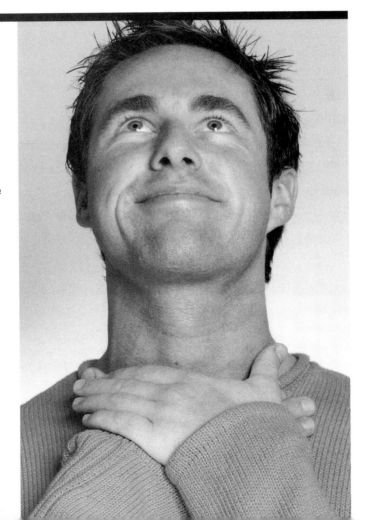

Facebuilder in the car

Because it's important for you to achieve your goals and because I know most of you have busy schedules, I've adapted all of the exercises so that you can do them in your car while driving home, to work, to the gym or wherever. All the exercises can be done easily and safely while driving, except for the Eye Toner and the Lower Eyelid Lift **which must only be practiced at a red traffic light or while the car is stationary**. Be careful and make sure you watch traffic lights and are aware of other vehicles.

Remember: Do not endanger yourself or others. Take great care while you are doing Facebuilding exercises in the car even while driving at very low speeds.

Car exercise 1 **Eye Toner**

Do this while waiting for the lights to change or when you are stationary. Place your index fingers between your brows and position your thumbs at your outer-eye corners. Forcefully squint up with the lower eyelid. Now hold the squint while squeezing your eyes shut tightly. Count to forty, then release. If you are at a traffic light, have a quick peep with one eye every few seconds to see if the light has changed.

Car exercise 2 **Lower Eyelid Lift**

This is an ideal exercise for when you are stationary, for example if you are stuck in traffic. Place your left thumb at the outer corner of your left eye and your left index finger at the outer corner of your right eye. Squint up strongly with your lower eyelids and hold the squint. Count to forty while keeping your upper eyelids wide open. Then place your thumb and index finger at your inner-eye corners. Squint up and then hold for a count of forty. Relax.

Car exercise 3 **Eyebrow Lift**

Place the thumb and index finger of one hand above each brow, in the middle of the forehead and pull your fingers down so that they are above your brows. Push your eyebrows up and release five times. Then hold your brows up, keeping the fingers pulled down. You'll feel a band of pressure build up across your forehead. Hold and count to twenty while pushing away on your steering wheel with the other hand. This movement intensifies the energy.

Car exercise 4 **Face Toner**

Place the thumb and index finger of one hand on top of each cheek. Open your mouth and pull your upper and lower lips away from each other, thus forming a long, strong, oval shape. Keep the long oval shape of the mouth strong—that's important. Also keep your upper lip pressed down firmly against your teeth. Smile with your mouth corners and then release. Repeat twenty-five times. Each time you should feel your cheek muscles move under your fingers. Use the power of your imagination to visualize the muscles pushing up under your cheeks. Also, each time you smile, with your other hand, push the steering wheel away and then release to intensify the energy. On the twenty-fifth smile, forcefully pull the upper and lower lip away from each other. Slowly move your thumb and index finger off your cheeks and up towards the roof of the car as you visualize the sides of your face lifting. Keep your upper and lower lips pulled away from each other. Hold and count to forty. Relax and blow out between your lips (see p. 51).

Car exercise 5 **Nose Toner**

Use your index finger to push the tip of your nose up and hold it firmly in place. Flex your nose down by pulling your upper lip down over your teeth. Hold this position for a second before releasing the lip. Repeat thirty-five times. You should feel the tip of your nose push against your finger each time.

Car exercise 6 **Mouth Toner**

Press your upper and lower lips together, focusing on the center of the lips. *Do not* purse them. Also be sure *not* to clench your teeth. Push your chin muscle up with your index finger and push against the steering wheel with your other hand. This will intensify the resistance and increase the benefit of the exercise. Hold the position until you can feel a burn in the center of your lips, then count to thirty. Relax and blow out between your lips (see p. 51).

Car exercise 7 **Smile Line Eraser**

Pull your upper and lower lips away from each other to make a long, strong, oval shape. Visualize a line of energy, moving from your mouth corners up to the sides of your nostrils. Use your thumb and index fingers to follow this line upward. Next, visualize that energy beam moving back down that imaginary line towards your mouth corners. Keep repeating this energy movement up and down, using your thumb and index finger to follow and intensify the energy. Do this exercise until you feel the burn, push away on the steering wheel, then pulse your thumb and index finger up and down for a count of thirty. Relax.

Car exercise 8 **Jaw Toner**

Open your mouth and roll your lower lip in tightly over the lower teeth. Pull the corners of your mouth toward your back teeth and roll them in tightly. Keep your upper lip pressed down firmly against the teeth. Place your index finger on your chin for resistance. Open and close your jaw in a slow, scooping motion using the corners of your mouth, not your jaw hinge. Push away on the steering wheel each time you scoop. Continue scooping until you feel the lactic acid burn. When you feel the burn, hold your jaw still in this pose and continue pushing on the steering wheel while counting to thirty. Then relax.

Car exercise 9 **Face Strengthener**

Open your mouth and pull the corners towards your back teeth, rolling them in tightly. Keep your upper lip firmly pressed down against your teeth. Visualize big fat cheeks coming out of the corners of the mouth. Position your thumb and index finger at the corners of your mouth and make small circular motions on your face. This will help you to mentally "expand" the sides of your face. Continue making the small, circular motions until you begin to feel the muscle widen. When this happens, slowly pull the fingers away from your face while continuing the circular motions. At the same time with the other hand push against the steering wheel for additional intensity. When you begin to feel the lactic acid burn in the sides of your face, make rapid circles with your fingers to intensify and enhance the energy. Count to thirty before relaxing. Relax and blow out between your lips.

Car exercise 10 **Facelift**

Open your mouth and forcefully roll your lips over your teeth. Pull the corners of your mouth toward your back teeth and roll them in tightly. Now visualize the sides of your face moving up and outward, past the jawline, to the top of the head. Push your face forward and your shoulders back. Continue moving this mental energy up along the sides of the face until you feel the burn, then push away from the steering wheel. Hold that position and count to thirty-five before releasing.

Car exercise 11 **Double Chin Toner**

Sit up straight with your chin held up high. Take care not to hold your chin so high, however, that you disrupt your line of vision. Close your lips and smile with your upper lip. Place one hand at the base of your throat, over the collarbone and pull down slightly on the skin. Tilt your head *slightly* backward and forward. You'll experience a strong pull on the chin and neck muscles. Tilt your head backward and forward thirty-five times.

6

Skincare basics and antiaging

For most men, skincare is still pretty basic. You shave, hop in the shower, lather up, wash your face with shower soap and you're off and running. Well, for all you twentieth-century guys out there, here's an update from the twenty-first century. Unless you want to look like a walking slab of beef jerky, you're going to have to take *much* better care of your skin than you probably have been doing. Your skin does a great job of taking care of you. Don't you think it's time you did the same for your skin, especially the skin on your neck and face? When you finish reading this chapter you're definitely going to *want* to take better care of your skin, especially the skin that shows the most.

Most of us are born with normal healthy skin, but genetics and lifestyle choices can dramatically compromise both our own and our skin's well-being as we age. What you put into your body, as well as how you treat it, influences your skin's health, color and texture. While some of us obviously have a healthier lifestyle than other people, it's never too late to improve the health and vitality of your skin. An old Buddhist saying states that the human body is a temple: Don't desecrate it.

Facebuilder is the key to help you unlock a youthful appearance, but there are other things you can do, in conjunction with the exercises, that will accelerate the progress towards the youthful appearance you want (and can definitely have). This chapter will outline some of the things necessary for a healthy lifestyle program.

In case you haven't noticed, the grooming that women have been practicing for centuries is now catching on big time with men. Men who belong to "Generation X," "Generation Y," the "New Generation," the "Me, Me Generation," the "Baby Boomers"—you name it—are all jumping aboard the Grooming Express in droves. And there are plenty of products at their disposal now. Skincare lotions, haircare products, antiaging supplements, bodycare products and tanning lotions all designed specifically for men are now widely available. Many men are now aware of the fact that if you want to make it big, you have to make a big effort.

Skin specifics

The skin is truly an amazing organ. It's like an ever-vigilant bodyguard, tirelessly standing watch over the body's well-being around the clock. Overworked and under-appreciated, it relentlessly filters out dirt and toxins in the air. It also does its best to ward off the sun's dangerous radiation. It comprises about 15 percent of our total body weight. The approximate chemical composition of the skin (for anyone who's getting ready to go on a quiz show) is as follows: water 70 percent, protein 25.5 percent, lipids 2 percent, trace minerals 0.5 percent and everything else about 2 percent.

How the skin ages

In the medical and scientific communities, there is no question that the way we treat the skin on our faces ages us more quickly than the actual aging process itself. A good case in point is that ubiquitous cowboy, the Marlboro Man. He's spent years and years in the sun. You *know* he doesn't use a sunscreen. He wouldn't be caught dead using a sunscreen. He looks lined and weather-beaten and the skin on his face resembles the leather on his belt and saddle. He's spent most of his life abusing his skin and he's got more wrinkles than he has cows in his herd. Trust me, he didn't get those "wrinks" from sleeping with his face in a pillow. He got them from mistreating his face. Marlboro Man is an excellent example of *extrinsic* (external) aging. In fact, he should be the poster boy for extrinsic aging.

You may not be quite so tanned, but you can see the effects the sun has by having a quick glance at the areas of your body which seldom or never get sun exposure, for example your bottom and upper thighs. Check out the difference between those areas and your lower arms, hands, upper chest and facial areas. Notice the difference? Of course you do. The areas most exposed are showing the most visible signs of aging.

We also have to contend with what is called *intrinisc* (internal) aging—nature's reward for growing older. As we age, our bodies are less resilient than when we were younger. It's common sense. Think about a nice shiny new car. You wax it when you bring it home (or have it waxed because you're busy). You wax it several times a year but after a few years, some areas of the car are beginning to fade a little. The hood, the roof and the trunk lid, for example. These are the areas that get the most direct sunlight. If the sun's rays can find their way through all that wax to do a number on the paint, think about what they are capable of doing to the skin of your face.

We're bombarded daily with information pertaining to exercise, diet, health and antiaging. The overwhelming amount of information out there is just too much for most of us to process and assimilate. So, let's simplify and condense here. In a nutshell, there are six major areas that you need to be concerned with if your goal is to maintain a youthful look long-term. They are:

■ Sun sense
■ Nutrition and supplements
■ Exercise

■ Sleep and stress management
■ Basic skincare
■ Grooming

Sun sense

Practicing preventative skin maintenance is paramount if you want to maintain a healthy, youthful complexion. It is essential even at a young age, because today's poor lifestyle choices will inexorably lead to tomorrow's skin disasters. Skin, being an external organ, is naturally exposed to the outside elements. Because of this, it ages faster than any other organ of the body. Some skin areas age much faster than other areas, however, because of overexposure to extrinsic conditions such as pollution, the weather and the sun.

Remember the song, "Here Comes The Sun," by George Harrison? The follow-up should be "Look What It's Done To My Skin, Ma." Our skin is super-susceptible to many things, but the most hostile element it will ever encounter is the sun. The sun supercharges the normal aging process: it is truly a skin "assassin." It's silent, surreptitious, incredibly patient, and it can be lethal. Strong words, you say? The sun is healthy, you think to yourself. A tan is attractive and desirable. Let's tell it like it is. Scientists and the medical community estimated that 90 percent of what we think of as signs of age are actually signs of overexposure to sunlight. Skin cancers kill over 100,000 people a year in the U.S. and over 50 percent of Americans over the age of sixty-five will experience at least one bout of skin cancer. There are over one million new skin cancer patients emerging every year in the U.S. alone, and many millions more worldwide. According to Martin A. Weinstock M.D., chief dermatologist at Providence, RI Veterans Affairs Medical Center in the U.S., "Skin cancer is now about as common as all other cancers combined." And, unfortunately, there's no evidence that the epidemic has peaked. Actually, there's no reason to assume that it will *ever* peak, given the gradual thinning and eroding of the earth's protective ozone layer year after year.

Tanning

UV (ultraviolet) radiation from the sun is the main cause of skin cancer. To complicate matters, there are several types of UV rays. UVA rays (the aging rays) penetrate deep into the skin, causing certain skin allergies as well as premature wrinkling. UVB rays (the burning rays) don't have the skin penetrative ability that UVA rays do, but they burn the skin, which triggers the body's defense mechanism to produce melanin and rush it to the skin's surface. Melanin is the pigment that darkens the skin to protect it, in effect creating a tan. It's ironic that the body knows what's best for itself and designs tactics to ward off danger while the owners of the bodies don't have the same common sense. A great many people constantly put their bodies in harm's way due to ignorance or possibly just due to an attitude that "a little bit of this and a little bit of that won't hurt me." Wrong. Hurt isn't a strong enough word to use here. Try *big* or *mega-hurt*. Better yet, use the word *destroy*.

It's vitally important to remember that we can be damaged by UV radiation from devices such as sun lamps and tanning booths. We have all been conditioned to admire a tan and many people still believe it is healthy and attractive. In fact, a tan is exactly the opposite of healthy and attractive. Our ancestors knew that. They covered up big time. Having a tan back in the old days was not considered cool at all. In fact it was considered lacking in refinement and a symbol of being lower class. After all, only the lower classes earned a living toiling in the sun. Being as tan-free as possible was prestigious. Not any more, apparently. The image of sun-tanned individuals, looking healthy and prosperous, probably originated in Hollywood in the 1940s and that image has really taken hold and is hard to shake. I'm always totally blown away when someone tells me that they are going to a tanning booth because they don't have time to sit in the sun or go to the beach. It's like they're saying, "I want to really damage my skin and I want to do it *now*." It's almost like standing in front of a microwave oven, shouting, "Hurry up. Hurry up." How quick do you want it?

Tanning booths and the sun both inflict the same type of UV destruction on the skin. Tanning booths just fast-forward the process. Both sources thicken the skin on a permanent basis, a process the medical community refers to as photoaging. This *absolutely* needs to be avoided if you don't want to end up in your dermatologist's office, having skin cancers zapped off your face. That's your best case scenario. That and wrinkles. The worst case scenario would be ending up as a morbid statistic—one of the many thousands of men who shoot through each year from skin cancer.

Sun damage

The intrusive penetration of UV rays cause the cosmetic ravaging we call aging. The rays of the sun continually unleash molecular mutants called "free radicals," which I discuss in depth on page 93. The sun's rays also wreak havoc on the proteins that normally keep your skin smooth, flexible and strong. This carnage results in all the things we associate with aging, namely: dry, wrinkled, sagging uneven skin, discoloration, age spots and an excellent chance of developing some type of skin disorder that could lead to basal cell carcinomas (slow-growing skin cancers), squamous cell carcinomas (faster-moving skin cancers) or melanomas (turbo-charged skin cancers that can quickly spread to other organs of the body, often with fatal results).

Basal and squamous cell cancers originate on the areas of the skin most exposed to the sun. The face, head, neck, arms and hands are the most common sites for these abnormalities. However, it should be noted that skin cancers can occur anywhere on the body. That's why you should see your family doctor immediately if you spot any kind of new mole or detect a change in an existing one. You should do this even if you have not been a sun worshipper. You should be particularly watchful if you're fair-skinned with light-colored eyes. Remember also that virtually all skin cancers can be cured if they are discovered and brought to a dermatologist's attention before they've had a chance to grow and spread. Be vigilant. It could save your life.

Here are several sun sense suggestions for protecting your skin:

1. Avoid the most harmful rays by staying out of the sun at least between the hours of 10am and 3pm. You don't have to be sunbathing to get mega doses of sun damage. Over 70 percent of sun damage to the skin is incurred during common, everyday activities such as driving and walking to and from your car.

2. Always wear a protective layer of sunscreen with at least a minimum SPF thirty rating to ward off UV radiation.

3. Always protect your face with a wide-brimmed hat and wear polarized sunglasses designed to protect your eyes from the harmful UV radiation. It's also a very good idea to wear a loose, lightweight long-sleeved shirt and long trousers when out in the sun. It may not be the Tommy Bahama image you'd like to project, but it sure beats going to the doctor later down the line with serious skin disorders.

Nutrition and supplements

Just about every girl I've ever known has been on a diet at one time or another and they don't work. Totie Fields once said, "I've been on a diet for two weeks and all I lost is two weeks." I love that saying. How many of you guys have tried to lose a few pounds and didn't lose anything, especially not your appetite? We all need to keep the following in mind: Balanced nutrition and exercise are both vital ingredients for a healthy lifestyle. Speaking of nutrition and exercise reminds me of something I observed not too long ago when I was at my gym. I saw a man wolfing down a big bagel in the snack bar. Fifteen or twenty minutes later, I saw the same fellow on the treadmill, sweating up a storm. He obviously was not aware of the fact that his body wouldn't be dipping into his stored body fat until every last gram of carbohydrate (his big bagel contained over 300 calories—all carbs) had been burned up. This translates into that man being on the treadmill until the cows come home, dripping sweat, wringing wet and wondering why his love handles weren't getting any smaller. Exercising is important but you have to remember to eat smart, too. Either one without the other won't get the job done.

Fat and sugar: The facts

We may not like this fact, but it's estimated that each and every one of us is born with more than twenty-three billion fat cells. These fat cells can get bigger when we eat the wrong kinds of foods. They can also get smaller if we eat the right kinds of foods, so what we eat is paramount to proper weight stabilization. Everyone needs some fat in their diet, but even those of us who actually do try to regulate the fat we eat get way too much from hidden sources. We need to ferret out the hidden fats and sugars our fat cells love to store.

No one who is serious about a healthy lifestyle would purposely eat the wrong foods because they are aware that this will accelerate weight gain and the aging process as well as sabotage their health and fitness program. However, many of us are consuming too much fat and sugar *unknowingly*. There are some very well-hidden fats and sugars in the most unlikely places. It's not just Coke that contains lots of calories, for example. Fructose (fruit sugar) occurs naturally in fruit and is generally considered to be a healthy substance. However, one 8 oz. glass of orange juice contains about 30 grams of sugar and over 135 calories. Drinking too much fruit juice on a regular basis can wreak havoc with your diet.

Cereals can be another source of sugar, along with breads and pastries. Eat enough of these items and you'll end up making the Pillsbury Doughboy look anorexic. And the next time you're prowling the supermarket, check out some of those "fat-free" cakes and cookies you've been loading up on lately. Read the labels on the packets. They may be lower in fat, but they are hardly fat free. And what about those low-fat meats in the deli section? They may be lower in fat than the standard version, but a horrifying number of their calories are still derived from fat. Also, you need to be wary of milk. The medical community used to say that you should drink at least three glasses of milk a day. Not any more. Milk may be healthy and you see athletes and celebrities endorsing it, with their cute little milk moustaches, but you won't slim down if you drink it, even if you drink the low fat variety.

Good nutrition

A diet high in fat, salt or sugary foods denies the body the nutrients it needs to effectively build muscle as well as to generate the energy and enthusiasm necessary for doing Facebuilder exercises. A typical Western diet also quickly adds unsightly bulges in various, mostly highly visible, body locations and, as a result, the second fastest-growing plastic-surgery procedure for men is liposuction. There has been around a four-fold increase in the number of liposuctions taking place in the U.S. since 1992. If your goal in life is to become a frequent fixture in a plastic surgeon's office, saying hello to his cannula or laser on a regular basis, then keep loading up on the salt, fat and sugar. Just don't forget that liposuction surgery is not much fun, for you or your wallet.

However, if your goal is to build strong, supportive facial and body muscles and to gain a smooth, clear complexion while seriously slowing down the aging process, you need to become aware of nutrition. The significance of a balanced diet is that it provides the body with the essential nutrients it needs daily, including vitamins, minerals and trace elements.

You should eat one to two portions of good-quality protein each day. Choose lean chicken, turkey, fish, beef or eggs. Protein is needed for growth and repair of the connective tissues within the skin. Vegetables and fruits high in fiber are always a safe choice for a healthy lifestyle, so try to eat five portions a day. The vitamins and minerals in fresh fruits and veggies are great for feeding your skin and for assisting your body in building and repairing cells. Many nutritional studies support the findings that vitamins C, E and A, plus minerals such as selenium and zinc, help to combat the breakdown of collagen and elastin, the skin's supporting and connective tissues.

As well as avoiding foods that contain saturated fats or sugars whenever you can, you should also exercise caution when seasoning food with salt. Salt makes your body retain water and can make your face and body puff up big time. Try to remember that the two main ingredients in salt (sodium and chloride) are deadly to the human body by themselves. Fortunately they neutralize each other when they come together to form salt. You can substitute herbs and spices in place of salt for flavoring and you will get more than enough salt in your daily diet to satisfy your body's requirements without adding one single shake of salt to your food. Keep that in mind when you have the salt shaker in your hand.

Water

"Water, water everywhere, nor any drop to drink," cried the Ancient Mariner in Samuel Coleridge's marathon poem. The Mariner was out in the ocean, low on drinking water, in deep trouble and he knew it. He no doubt was aware of the fact that water is a fundamental element of human life. It is the universal solvent, aiding in digestion and absorption of food. It also carries nutrients and oxygen to every cell in our body, while flushing out toxins and other wastes.

Water offers the body numerous benefits, including the following:
- Suppressing the appetite
- Assisting in the metabolism of stored fat
- Reducing fat deposits in the body
- Relieving fluid retention
- Reducing sodium build-up
- Maintaining proper muscle tone
- Ridding the body of wastes and toxins
- Relieving constipation
- Regulating the body's cooling system.

Consuming at least eight glasses of water a day has been a mantra for many years, and for good reason. Drinking this amount of water will help to keep your skin clear and assist in keeping your muscles and skin toned and healthy. In spite of a few unfortunate, highly publicized deaths of athletes due to dehydration, most well-informed coaches and sportsmen know that nobody should avoid fluids while exercising. In fact hydration is absolutely vital for peak performance. When you exercise, you must be well hydrated because water is needed to store glycogen, the fuel muscles require to convert protein into new muscle. Plenty of water is also needed to keep the body reasonably cool during exercise. Water transports electrolytes (the dissolved chemicals that carry electrical messages between the nerves and muscles) and it lubricates the joints. Without enough water, muscles will shrink in size, the nerve signals will scramble, nutrients will reach their destination more slowly, muscle contractions will weaken and the result will be that athletic performance is compromised.

You literally are what you drink. All you guys should develop a "drinking plan" and I'm not talking about the one you probably put into effect in college. Here are some suggestions for a *sensible* water-drinking plan.

1. As a minimum, try to drink eight glasses every day. Studies have shown repeatedly that if you are overweight, according to the average height and weight comparison charts, you should drink one extra glass of water for every twenty-five pounds you carry over your recommended weight.

2. Try bottled mineral water, which contains fewer toxins than tap water in most areas of the country, and is healthier for you.

3. Drink one or two glasses of water when you wake up in the morning and another one or two just before you go to bed.

4. Keep a couple of bottles of water on your desk and try to drink them during the day.

5. Remember that it's better to drink water cold. It's absorbed more quickly and it's supposed to burn more calories this way.

6. If you aren't drinking enough water, your body will begin to retain water to com-

pensate for what it intuitively knows to be water shortage. To eliminate fluid retention, drink more water, not less.

7. Make a conscious effort to skip the Cokes, fruit juices and cups of tea and coffee
whenever possible. They are "water bandits" who steal large quantities of water from
the body in order to facilitate their own digestion.

8. It's also important to steer clear of alcohol. Sorry to be the party pooper here, but
alcohol acts as a diuretic and actually accelerates body fluid loss. This results in dehydration, which is the main cause of a hangover. When you do drink alcohol, drink
plenty of water, too.

9. Don't drink water thirty minutes before, during or after a meal. Water dilutes the
digestive process.

The bottom line is that water is the single most important nutrient you take in each
and every day. It's fat-free, cholesterol-free, low in sodium, calorie free and it tastes
great.

Antiaging supplements

Before I talk about antiaging supplements, I believe that everyone needs to be familiar
with a theory proposed in 1954 by Dr. Denham Harmon, which is almost universally
accepted by the medical community today. Dr. Harmon's theory goes directly to the
heart of the aging process, which occurs in every human being. He stated that the
body contains what he called "free radicals." These unfriendly little atoms or groups of
atoms are created, in part, by the way our cells utilize oxygen to produce energy.
Free radicals are unstable oxygen molecules created during the body's basic metabolic
functions, such as digestion and breathing. All these little guys have one thing in common. They contain at least one unpaired electron. This creates a problem. If an electron is unpaired, another molecule or atom can hook up with it. This "bonding"
creates a chemical reaction that may not always be positive. Picture someone hook-

ing up with someone else after a few drinks at a cocktail party. Maybe it's a right match. Maybe not. Free radicals don't have a long life-span either. Maybe just a split second. However, that's enough time for them to do some serious damage to neighboring cells when these "bondings" are mismatched.

So, what does all this scientific information have to do with aging, you may ask? It has *everything* to do with aging. These unholy alliances cause reactions that are speculated to contribute to heart muscle cell damage, nerve cell damage, cancer, hardening of the arteries and a host of other degenerative disorders that may number as many as eighty at the time of writing. Dr. Harmon's studies ironically pinpointed one of life's great paradoxes. Most free radicals are oxygen-based. We need oxygen to sustain life, yet oxygen promotes free radicals, which cause aging and disease. If it's not one thing, it's the same thing, as I like to say.

Another paradox is that not all free radicals are harmful to our bodies. There are some that are definitely beneficial because they can help destroy the viruses and bacteria that attack our bodies. They also help to produce some very necessary hormones and enzymes that are vital to human life. *Most* free radicals are *not* beneficial to us, however, and we need to do all we can to avoid overwhelming our body with these inadvertently hostile invaders.

It's bad enough that our own bodies manufacture these mutants but it gets worse. Factors such as air pollution, radiation and sunlight, not to mention cigarette smoke from other people, all create free radicals. If you smoke, or associate with people who smoke, you need to be aware of the horrendously toxic elements in cigarette smoke. Remember, these toxic elements contribute to the proliferation of free radicals.

I discuss the prolific dangers of tanning on page 82, but it bears mentioning again here. When we are out in the sun, unprotected, even for a very short period of time, molecules in the skin absorb sunlight. Once these molecules are activated they turn into free radicals almost immediately. They then turn on their neighbor molecules as described above. Free radicals attack and injure vital cell structures such as collagen and cellular membranes. These attacks can leave small defects in the skin that eventually turn into wrinkles. Again, I cannot stress this enough: For your skin's sake, stay out of the sun and avoid cigarette smoke whenever possible.

Antioxidants

What can we do about free radicals? This is a good question. Fortunately, there are certain nutrients known as antioxidants, which have proven extremely effective in slowing down or even reversing the ravages of the free radical assault on our bodies. Antioxidants are compounds that aid the body in disarming the free radicals, so to speak. They are instrumental in helping our bodies deactivate or at least minimize the free radical ravages within our cells. These antioxidant warriors can prevent free radicals from running amok in the body by giving these mutant molecules new electrons to replace the ones they've lost. Once the antioxidant hooks up with the free radical, the free radical is stabilized and ceases its pilfering activity against neighbor cells. The antioxidant actually neutralizes the free radical and renders it harmless. Antioxidants can also help repair sun-related damage caused by free radicals and they may even help reduce the risk of skin cancers.

It's important to note here that Dr. Harman was the first to illuminate the free radical problem, but another doctor named Imre Nagy expanded on Dr. Harman's theory. Dr. Nagy agreed with Dr. Harman that free radicals were the primary causes of age-related problems, but he went a step further. He suggested that most of the aging damage was experienced by the outer layers of the cell. Prior to Dr. Nagy's theory, most scientists and dermatologists believed that primary free radical damage was experienced by the interior of the cell, causing cellular DNA damage and, hence, aging. But Dr. Nagy was able to prove that DNA extracted from the cells of elderly people, even those over ninety years old, was able to reproduce normally. Since the DNA was not damaged, DNA damage could not be the primary cause of aging. From the findings culminating from Dr. Nagy's research, scientists have been able to develop antioxidants that are designed to penetrate cell membranes, aid in the repair of these cells and increase their ability to retain water, which is vital to the cell's well-being. Without water, the cell becomes dehydrated. The work of these two doctors, among others, has proven invaluable in the development of treatments which appear to help reverse the signs of aging.

So where do we find these antioxidants? Here is a list of some of the top antioxidants and their sources:

■ **Selenium** Top foods containing selenium include seafood, meat, Brazil nuts, tuna, wholegrains, cottage cheese and chicken. As well as having antioxidant properties, selenium also seems to help relieve anxiety: In one university college study most of the men and women who took a daily dose of 100mg of selenium for just five weeks reported feeling less anxious, less depressed and less tired.

■ **Betacarotene** Orange and dark-green vegetables, such as spinach, carrots and sweet potatoes, are rich sources of betacarotene. High levels of this antioxidant seem to cut the risk of lung, mouth, throat, oesphagus, larynx, stomach, breast and bladder cancer.

■ **Vitamin C** This can be found in all fruit and vegetables but particularly good sources are citrus fruits, broccoli, green and red peppers and strawberries. The Nobel Prize-winning scientist Linus Pauling, who lived to be ninety-three, stated that we could add twelve to eighteen more years to our lives by taking 3,200 to 12,000mg of vitamin C a day.

■ **Vitamin E** Nuts and seeds, including peanuts, almonds, sunflower and sesame seeds, and wheatgerm are all rich in vitamin E. Dr. Eric Rimm, author of a Harvard study on the role of vitamin E in the prevention of heart disease, said, "The risk of not taking vitamin E is equivalent to the risk of smoking."

■ **Other antioxidants** Vitamin B12, vitamin A, folic acid and pycnogenol are also beneficial antioxidants. Pycnogenol, which is an extract of pine bark, is considered to be the most powerful antioxidant available at the time of writing, and it has proven extremely effective against environmental toxins. Research indicates that pycnogenol is twenty times stronger than vitamin C. It also activates vitamin C and gets it working hard before it leaves your body.

Oxidative stress

Since we know that antioxidants can disarm and render free radicals harmless, and we know that free radicals are the primary cause of aging, then why do we age at all? Here's why. Our everyday exposure to the sun, cigarette smoke and other noxious pollutants creates a constant barrage of new free radicals. It's this inexorable onslaught of newly created free radicals that can overwhelm the antioxidant army, allowing these newcomer mutants to move about our bodies at will, creating more and more free radicals. Scientists refer to this phenomenon (the constant creation of new free radicals) as *oxidative stress* and it goes on *ad infinitum*. The good news here is that we can slow down the rate of carnage the free radicals inflict on our bodies by taking supplements and exercising common sense. The bad news is that scientists are not yet able to completely reverse oxidative stress and that is why our bodies continue to age, despite all of our precautions.

We shouldn't be discouraged at the prospect of oxidative stress. But we do need to take supplements and eat vitamin-rich foods. These substances give our bodies a tremendous advantage in the war against aging. **Caution:** Because everyone's biochemistry is unique, it would be prudent for you to consult a nutritionist before embarking on any antioxidant supplement program.

Exercise

Oxygen is crucial to life. The normal human body can survive for weeks without food (and many should). It can also survive for days without water. But it can't survive for more than a few minutes without oxygen—truly this substance is the staff of life. Apart from being essential for the production of energy, oxygen is vital for synthesizing fats, proteins, carbohydrates and other substances in food, thereby helping to build and maintain cells, organs, muscles, bones and other structures.

Oxygen is important for a clear skin and the most effective way to increase your oxygen intake is to exercise at least three times a week. Exercise definitely makes you look and feel better. After a good workout, your skin will take on a healthy, vital glow. Aerobic exercises such as jogging or spinning (bike riding) increase blood circulation which, in turn, enhances the flow of oxygen and nutrients to all parts of your body, including your skin. Clinical studies conducted in various countries throughout the world have proven, beyond any doubt, that aerobic exercise (elevating the heart and breathing rates to higher than average levels) for thirty minutes or more, at least three times a week, will keep you healthier and more fit. It's also a tremendous stress buster (for all you workaholics out there).

Physical activity greatly benefits the skin by increasing the flow of blood and oxygen throughout the skin tissue and it also introduces oxygen and other nutrients, needed for the maintenance and repair of the skin cells. Oxygenated blood helps remove toxins and internal pollutants, which can otherwise damage the skin and connective tissues. When you exercise to the point where you make your skin flush, you can see the color of your skin change. This is a result of the oxygenated blood, coursing vigorously throughout your body, replenishing and repairing as it goes. If you are not in great shape, even mild exercise such as a brisk thirty-minute walk will help get your blood pumping and will give your skin a healthy, robust appearance. **Caution:** If you are over forty or have not exercised recently, it is always prudent to seek the approval of your doctor before initiating any kind of exercise program.

Deep breathing

Deep breathing is a mild, but effective, form of exercise. Like the Facebuilder exercises, it can be done anywhere. You can do it while driving, sitting at your desk, waiting for the lift, or pretty much in any situation. Deep breathing will make your heartbeat accelerate initially, pumping more oxygenated blood through your body. Like an internal massage, deep yogic breathing will bring on a calm, energized feeling. It is exceptionally effective if you're feeling stressed because you have an important presentation to make or a big meeting with your boss, or even because you happen to be a highly wired kind of person. Most politicians and public speakers with whom I've come in contact have told me that they do deep breathing before an important speech or presentation to calm and center themselves.

Most of the time we take short shallow breaths, utilizing only the upper portion of our lungs. Deep breathing means breathing from your diaphragm located in your stomach area. You literally have to teach yourself the art of deep breathing. Here's how you do it. Sit up straight with your shoulders relaxed. Do not lean forward. Inhale through your nose. Slowly fill your lungs with a deep breath. Try to expand your lower ribcage as you inhale. Eventually, you should feel the air moving into the top of your lungs. When you've reached maximum breathing capacity (when it feels like you're going to pop), hold your breath for ten full seconds. Then slowly exhale through your mouth. Relax and breathe normally for four breaths. Repeat this procedure ten times. It definitely works—try it.

Sleep and stress management

When the Irish poet James Stephens said, "Sleep is an excellent way of listening to the opera," he was only partially correct. Sleep is absolutely vital for human beings to survive (especially if you don't like opera) and it has many beneficial effects.

Everyone knows how revitalized and refreshed we feel after a good night's sleep. That's partly why bed time is many a man's favorite time of day. What many people *don't* know is that sleep is also a very good refresher and nourisher of the skin. Scientists call lack of sleep "sleep deprivation." I call it a "nocturnal bandit," robbing you of the essential rest and recuperation your skin needs to look its best throughout your life.

When you don't get enough sleep, your face will pay the price. Your reward for skipping sleep is a tired, sagging face. Without sleep your system begins to shut down, it doesn't just request sleep—it demands it. Without sleep, muscles become fatigued and the face will begin to droop and sag, or worse. The skin begins to take on a sallow, dull appearance. Then, other problems start to develop. The blood pressure and the pulse begin to drop. This results in less blood and oxygen being pumped to the facial area. In short, you aren't going to be looking so hot. People are going to think you look like you need to get some sleep, and they're right. International studies indicate that an alarming number of people (over 63 percent and rising) are sleep-deprived. Everyone should get at least seven to eight hours of sleep a night to look, feel and be your best. Anyone who says they can get by on less than seven hours of sleep a night probably has been and definitely looks like it. It wouldn't be so bad losing an extra hour or two of sleep here and there, if those hours were spent relaxing or working on a hobby, but studies show that those extra hours are increasingly being spent at the office, playing catch-up. The National Sleep Foundation has said "instead of working to live, more and more Americans are living to work." The Foundation goes on to say that this shift has a profound impact on personal lives. You bet it does. To quote NFS director Richard L. Gelula, "Statistically, it's been shown that people who sleep too little don't live so long." The last time I checked, no one on their deathbed ever said that they wished they'd spent more time at the office. Words to *live* by, guys.

Here are a few tips for a better night's sleep. Following them will add years to your life, so they are worth noting:
- Avoid caffeine for at least six hours before bedtime.
- Say *adios* to alcohol and nicotine for two hours before you hop into bed.
- Go to bed and get up at set times.
- Try to take a short nap sometime during the day. Even a twenty-minute "power nap" will improve your mental dexterity.
- Try to exercise for at least thirty minutes a day (but not late at night).
- Take a warm shower or bath an hour or so before going to bed.
- If you need a bedtime snack, eat turkey or dairy products. They contain tryptophan, a natural sleep-inducer.
- If you have trouble falling asleep, get up and do something dull. No TV, though. The bright light will tell your brain to stay awake, even if the show you're watching is dull.

Night-time skincare

One of the most common complaints I receive, on a daily basis it seems, is what I like to call the "wrinkles on the face when I wake up" syndrome. Some people are truly horrified when they glance in a mirror upon wakening. This is because many people sleep with their face in the pillow. They don't start off sleeping that way, but because of night-time tossing and turning, they end up face down in the pillow when they wake up. Most people don't think they move around that much during sleep, but studies have shown that many people gyrate quite a bit during the night.

We go through different stages as we sleep. We start out in a light sleep (the *theta* state). Then we enter the *delta* state, when we are in deep sleep. This is when your body is regenerating. Tension and the problems of the previous day are reduced to a minimum during this time. The deep sleep period doesn't last all that long, however. Within an hour or so, you enter another state, known as the Rapid Eye Movement (REM) stage. During this stage, your brain is functioning almost as though you are awake, but you're not. Your body remains asleep. Your mind is back at work, however, resolving problems, releasing thoughts, etc. We go through several stages of REM activity and this is good. The more REM sleep you get, the more likely you are to wake up feeling refreshed, energized and positive. During a normal seven- to eight-hour sleep span, you will probably have four or five REM sleep episodes. The last REM episodes last the longest and are the most beneficial, which is why getting seven to eight hours of sleep a night is so critical. Some people think they need less than seven hours' sleep. Not true. Others don't get the necessary hours because of lack of physical exercise, poor eating habits, consumption of alcohol or caffeine or disturbances during the night.

If you don't sleep well, you may have a tendency to start "tossing and turning," like Bobby Lewis sang in his song of the same name. It's this activity which puts you in the positions that may not be good for you over the course of a night's sleep. That's why some people wake up with their faces in a pillow, which will cause wrinkles. You can't control your dreams but you can control your sleeping position. You want to sleep on your back all night. A good habit to initiate is to sleep without a pillow under your head. While this may seem uncomfortable at first, it's the best way to get a good night's sleep without moving around all that much. You can use a neck roll, if you feel you need something but put that pillow under your knees and lay flat on your back when you fall asleep. This will be very beneficial to those of you who have a bad back because it'll keep your spine straight. Also, this will definitely cut down on your nocturnal gyrations and will result in a sound, healthy, beneficial good night's sleep. And you won't wake up looking like "pillowface."

Basic skincare

Before you can learn how to take care of your skin, you have to know what kind of skin you have. When it comes to skin types, most men are totally clueless as to what type of skin they have. They also are not aware that all types need care and attention.

I often have clients, for example, who will tell me that they don't think they need to use a moisturizer. They'll say, "I have oily skin." I tell them that even though their skin may be oily, they still need water because normal skin contains both of these elements. Skin types are classified into three categories—normal, oily and dry. Many people have a combination of the types. Skin type can change over the years so you need to be aware of this.

Normal skin

Normal skin has it all: good muscle tone, resiliency and optimum hydration. It appears soft, plump, moist and has a healthy color and glow. A great example of normal skin would be a child's skin, before puberty. As skin starts to age, however, it also starts to change. It could start to have less oil than it used to. I tell clients the reason for this occurrence is that they are probably losing moisture in their skin because they are using harsh cleansers, such as soap, to wash away the oil. Does that sound familiar, guys?

There are many factors at work which speed up the aging of the skin. One main culprit is lack of water. Many people think that if they drink soft drinks, tea, coffee, beer or alcoholic beverages, then they don't need to drink lots of water. The items mentioned above *do not* take the place of water, because the body processes them differently. For your skin's sake, you should drink at least eight glasses of water a day. You should also avoid harsh soaps, solar radiation and other environmental exposures, which all have an adverse effect on the skin.

Normal skin requires cleansing in the evening. We all need to be consistent in the use of protective moisturizers, as well as a transdermal sunscreen (one that penetrates the skin) with a minimum SPF rating of thirty during the day. It might not seem macho, but you *should* always apply moisturizer before you jump into bed. You probably won't, but it would be better for your face if you did. It's up to you.

Oily skin

Oily skin is usually hereditary and is the result of overactive sebaceous glands. It often can be recognized from its thick, shiny and somewhat slack appearance. Oily skin sometimes will appear to be dirty or neglected. The pores of the skin will probably appear to be enlarged, due to oil that is trapped in the follicles. There may be a few blemishes on the chin or forehead areas and the skin will feel oily to the touch.

Heat and humidity exacerbate oily skin problems. If you have oily skin and live in a hot or humid climate you will most probably find your skin becomes even more oily. Using skincare products such as harsh soaps, or making excessive use of astringents or scrubs can make oily skin worse. The use of exfoliating products, such as enzyme and botanical products, can help to regulate the oil and improve the look and texture of oily skin.

If you have oily skin, you must pay special attention to thorough (but gentle) cleansing morning and evening. Protective moisturizers containing humectants (substances that attract and hold water) will assist the skin in maintaining the suppleness and moisture it requires. And don't forget to wear sunscreen. A common misconception among people with oily skin is that they don't need this. Wrong. You need it for sure. And make sure it's a sunscreen with a minimum SPF rating of thirty.

Dry skin

People with dry skin have sebaceous glands that are underactive—they do not produce enough of the secretions required to properly moisturize the skin. Dry skin is also a by-product of the aging process. The body's activity slows down as we grow older and the oil-gland activity slows down as well. Problems with dry skin are intensified by exposure to the sun and improper skincare. Dry skin, lacking the necessary oil content, is unable to retain moisture, since oil in the skin acts as a natural barrier to moisture loss. The characteristics of dry skin include tight, thin skin with tiny, superficial lines. Pores are almost invisible and the skin appears scaly and flaky. This type of skin wrinkles easily.

Proper care for dry skin should include daytime and night-time protection, using rich moisturizers and sunscreen with a minimum SPF rating of thirty. Proper cleansing is also a must, but only cleanse once a day, preferably right before bedtime. Excessive cleansing will strip away whatever natural oils there are in the skin and further dehydrate it, exacerbating the problem. Use hydrating facial cleansers, not that bar of soap in your shower, to clean and soften your dry skin. I know you don't think it's cool for a man to be using these products, but you need to anyway. Hey, it's your face!

Grooming

Men seem to be responding to a society whose consumer culture is less and less forgiving toward those who are not young, trim and attractive. That's most probably because they're being bombarded with advertising images of trim, younger-looking hunks. More and more of you are hitting the spas and skincare salons to get facials, haircare, manicures and massages. Cosmetic companies are introducing macho-sounding campaigns for their men's care product lines. The result is a mushrooming of men's skin and haircare product sales. The latest statistics reveal that this type of marketing is increasing sales of these products by 11 percent a year. In 2001, the men's grooming market was worth over $6 billion. These numbers keep ballooning astronomically every year. You guys are learning what women have always known. Looking good takes time, effort and costs a few bucks.

Most of you guys aren't going to want to take the following step, but you should. It's a well-known fact that no skincare regime is complete without exfoliation (the clearing away of dead skin). Regular exfoliation with an enzyme mask will get rid of the old and bring in the new. Enzymes fall within a classification of proteins known as "dynamic proteins." They temporarily attach themselves to molecules. In doing so, the molecule becomes ionized, transformed into a positively or negatively charged particle. Enzyme skin-tighteners are protein enzymes that enter the skin and hydrolyze the dead tissue. When enzymes are rinsed and removed, the dead tissue will flood out of the skin. In my experience, the enzyme masks that work the best contain protein, RNA, L-lysine and proline. These cleanse and penetrate the skin to tighten the epidermis. A good enzyme mask will constrict, tone and tighten the skin while drawing out impurities from the pores as described above. Like I said before, many of you guys won't want to take this step, but you should know that lots and lots of your buddies are probably hitting skincare salons and spas in droves and having skin treatments as you're reading this. They just aren't telling you about it. You don't believe me? Well, let me bring you up to speed here. A very recent study found that 83 percent of the men surveyed stated that they were "actively" trying to improve their looks. By actively, they meant taking treatments and other measures to look better. Those activities included facials, hair coloring, manicures and even (gasp) waxing. One out of three skin treatments being performed today in the U.S. are being performed on men. Perhaps even your friends are having treatments. Remember that old song by Carly Simon, "You're So Vain"? Did she know your friends? Do you?

The skincare products that I have found to be most valuable in aiding the skin are transdermal (i.e., they penetrate the skin). This allows the active ingredients to be stored in the skin for a period of time, allowing them to favorably influence the functions of cells and glands located within the dermis. Your best bet for locating high quality transdermal products is to talk to your dermatologist or to a licensed beautician. Or you can get in touch with me (see p. 112).

Some cosmetic manufacturers claim that oxygen-bearing emulsions can actually penetrate the skin and bring other nutrients such as vitamins A and B directly into skin cells to perform repair work. Do you recall the discussion on oxygen (see p. 93), the great vehicle for producing energy and continuous rejuvenation of our bodies? Oxygen-bearing cosmetics are some of the most highly touted products in today's cosmetic markets. The main active ingredient in oxygen cosmetics is medical-grade hydrogen peroxide. Bacteria, which contribute to skin problems such as acne, cannot survive in an oxygen rich environment. This would seem to indicate that oxygen acts as an antibacterial agent whether on or in the skin.

The latest products

The cosmetics industry continues to introduce new skincare products that promise to "revolutionize" men and women's skincare. It's a mega-buck business now and many new antiage skincare ingredients are being bandied about. How do you know if they work or not? "It's *caveat emptor*," according to Dr. Richard Glogau, a San Francisco dermatologist, "Let the buyer beware." With this in mind, I'll explain what some of the new ingredients being introduced to the market can do for you—including the so-called "buzz ingredients" you might have heard about.

■ **Alpha-Hydroxy and Beta-Hydroxy** Available in prescription and nonprescription strengths, these acids remove dead skin cells, revealing newer, tauter skin.

■ **Antioxidants** This group of chemicals, which includes vitamins C and E, Coenzyme Q-10 and the enzyme superoxide dismutase, scoop up free radicals (see pages 91–93). Preliminary research indicates that they may have disease-fighting properties.

■ **Copper Peptide** This chemical supposedly aids rejuvenation of the skin and reduction of wrinkles.

■ **D-Boldine Extract** This ingredient is found in the leaves and bark of the boldo tree, which is indigenous to Chile. It has particularly potent antioxidant and anti-inflammatory properties, making it an excellent cell-protective ingredient.

■ **Fullerenes** Water-soluble fullerenes (carbon spheres shaped like a football) show intriguing potential for skincare. Much smaller than liposomes and nanosomes, they are building blocks for collagen, incredible carriers for skincare ingredients and, most importantly, they show promise to become potent free radical scavengers.

■ **Furfuryladenine** This is an anti-withering agent found in the leaves of green plants. Early studies indicate that it might help reduce signs of sun damage such as blotches, fine wrinkles and roughness of the skin.

■ **Heavy Water Deuterium Oxide** (D20) is a rare water found in a few saline lakes and in deep seawater. It feels and tastes like regular water, but it is sweeter. It is 10 percent heavier than ordinary water. The hydrogen portion of heavy water is twice as heavy as the hydrogen in ordinary water, hence the term. Being heavier helps it to resist evaporation and it dries out more slowly. This is what makes it an excellent addition to skincare products.

■ **Spin Traps** Just when it seemed as though free radicals were gaining the upper hand in the battle to age us all as fast as possible, scientists have discovered a new substance which allows them to assemble an A-Team to turn the tide in the battle against aging. These new team members, called spin traps, are intelligent antioxidants. They are nitrone-based substances that trap free radicals and examine them to determine how to most effectively prevent them from causing skin cell damage. They also appear to have anti-inflammatory benefits, which would make them a tremendous help for aging skin. Spin traps have enormous potential for helping skin stay healthy. I love these little creatures. They are the new superheroes, whose job it is to protect and preserve healthy skin.

A perspective

Even though scientists continue to level the playing field with new wonder substances, it's always going to be paramount to remember what I have been stressing throughout this book: *most of the signs of aging are the result of sun damage.* You simply *have* to stay out of the sun. If you are going to be outside, at least stay in the shade during peak sun hours and wear SPF factor thirty sunscreen even in the shade. Says Dr. Norman Levine, a University of Arizona dermatologist, "All the stuff that is sold in the drug stores pales in comparison to the use of sunscreens for the prevention of wrinkles."

A final word

Every exercise I have outlined, every tip I have discussed has been designed to benefit your skin and your face. I pamper my skin every day of my life because I am not going to be able to trade it in later for a newer, sleeker model. Bodies aren't like cars, guys. We can't lease a new body every three or four years. We have to play the hand we've been dealt, but we have options on which cards we keep and which ones we throw away. This is what Facebuilder is all about. The techniques I've discussed in this book will teach you how to play the game successfully and end up with a winning hand. The ball's in your court.

In the many, many years I've been advocating and teaching facial exercises, I've met many hundreds of thousands of people from all walks of life, throughout the world. I've watched them undergo truly remarkable, even miraculous, changes in their faces and their lives by incorporating these exercises into their daily life patterns. Ten minutes a day, twice a day is not a large investment of time out of anyone's daily routine. Small investments, prudently made, can yield truly spectacular dividends. After all, $7,000 invested in Microsoft or Dell Computers in 1990 was worth millions and millions of dollars nine years later. Was that "small" investment worth it? You be the judge.

My facial training career has taken me on a truly remarkable journey around the world. I've loved every minute of the journey, which continues on, for me anyway, forever. I used a quote in my first book, which is a favorite of mine. It's an old Buddhist/Chinese saying which states, "when the student is ready, the master appears." There are students all over the world who are ready now, and Facebuilder is ready for them. It's never too late to do something truly beneficial for you and your face. Remember, facial exercises increase your face value.

Whenever you need encouragement, revisit the before and after photos of the guys whom I've pictured in the book. Those dramatic photos should give you all the encouragement you need to stick with the program. If you need more motivation, read some of the testimonials I've reprinted from the thousands and thousands of letters I've received over the years from satisfied clients worldwide. Facial excercise changed their lives forever. They definitely changed mine. They can do the same for you. Always remember that if you *really* want something, you can achieve it. And above all, seeing yourself as you want to be is the key to personal growth.

Testimonials

These are some comments from male clients who have used my techniques to enhance and improve their lives and their looks. I hope their words will encourage you to persevere.

Dear Carole:

I have been dealing with intestinal lipodystrophy and have found your face exercises to be very beneficial in reshaping and filling in the hollowed out look in my face. With all the other complications to deal with, I appreciate your program and what it has done to help me look and feel better.

T. Barsten, San Francisco, California

Dear Carole:

I have been stricken with acoustic neuroma, which can cause partial facial paralysis. I saw your book on the acoustic neuroma website and decided to give the exercises a try. The symmetry of my face was restored and the numbness relieved. After reading what others have dealt with, your book is really life-changing.

J. Newman, Miami, Florida

Dear Carole:

I am a dedicated body builder. I work out at Gold's Gym six days a week. My body is hard, cut and strong. However, my face had a sunken and tired look to it. I started doing your exercises after seeing you on TV. In just three week's time my face had become stronger and wider. The sunken area was filled in. Now I can honestly say that my face looks as good as my body.

J. Olson, Los Angeles, California

Dear Carole:

I play saxophone in a band and I have been doing your exercises for several years. I have noticed a firmness in my lips and mouth area that wasn't there before I took up your exercise program. My mouth doesn't get tired like it used to. That's an added benefit. The biggest benefit is that I look a lot better now than I used to. Thanks, Carole. This song's for you.

D. Perkins, Nashville, Tennessee

Dear Ms. Maggio:

My face is my fortune. I'm an actor and how I look determines if I get my part or not. In this business, you have to stay young looking if you want to keep working. I have been doing your exercise program faithfully for about six months now and I can honestly say that I don't think I'll be going under the knife any time soon, unlike some of my fellow actors. Thanks for your program.

Jeremy M., London

Dear Carole:

You probably don't get a lot of letters from guys, but I want to write and tell you that I have been doing your exercises faithfully for ten months now and I can see a very distinct difference in my jawline and chin area. I'm fifty-four years old and until I bought your book I was kind of resigned to looking my age. I exercise regularly, but my gym exercises were not helping my face. In fact, I think I was starting to look older than my years. But not now. I guess I should tell my friends my secret, but I think I'll just let them wait and wonder what I'm doing that is working when what they are doing isn't.

You're great. I saw your infomercial recently and you look terrific.

Ben M., Chicago, Illinois

Dear Ms. Maggio:

I am a forty-eight-year-old egocentric male who has high cheekbones and chiseled features. Though I've always looked younger than my age, I was beginning to sag around the jawline and eye area, which caused me to start looking my age. I started using your facial exercises in January and within five months, I looked about twenty-seven years young. The lifting of my entire face has been amazing. My skin tone is better than it ever has been and my face has actually become more muscular and chiseled.

I truly wish I had taken a "before" picture to compare my results today. I applaud you for your impressive product and thank you for helping me take years off of my appearance.

M. P., Pittsburgh, Pennsylvania

Dear Carole:

I've had Bell's palsy for six months. I had seen several physicians but nothing they did or suggested really helped all that much. I still had the numbness and paralysis. I started doing your exercises after seeing you on TV. You mentioned that they might help, so I decided to give it a try. Nothing ventured, nothing gained, right? Well, to my surprise, the sagging on the left side of my face has firmed up and the numbness has really subsided. Amazing.

Thanks, Carole,

John MacDonald, Glasgow

Dear Carole:

I have been suffering from TMJ for several years. I feel like it's stress related. I started doing your exercises at the suggestion of my family dentist. I no longer have the complications from TMJ which is a real benefit, but a great side benefit is that I look younger now. My face tightened up in the process. I asked my dentist how he knew this would work. He said it worked for him.

Jerry Kinmann, Portland, Oregon

Dear Carole:

I'm a victim of age discrimination. I lost my job in the tech downturn in California. When I went out job hunting, I felt I was not getting offers I was qualified for. I dyed my hair back to black, lost some weight and (at my wife's suggestion) started doing your face exercises with her. I noticed a very quick improvement. I am now working again and I really believe that the way I look now helped me get my new job.

D. Hatcher, San Jose, California

Dear Carole:

I have used your facial exercise program for a year or so now. I was in a serious car accident two years ago and I broke many bones in my face, which left my face numb and disfigured. Your exercises restored the feeling and symmetry to my face. I was actually anticipating having to undergo several surgeries so this is just amazing for me.

Rick Griffin, Mobile, Alabama

Dear Carole:

My wife and I have been married for thirty years. Several years ago, we planned to attend a high school reunion. My wife was doing your face exercises because she wanted to look her best. I decided to give it a try. To make a long story short, we both looked a lot younger than our "old" friends. They all thought we'd both had face-lifts.

Paul Greggs, Seattle, Washington

Dear Carole:

My eyelids started to go south on me in my early forties. I couldn't afford the surgery I was told I would need to make things better. Your book and video were much less expensive. I've been doing the exercises for six months or so now and I can notice a big difference. My eyes are much more open now and I don't have the puffiness under the eyes that I had before I started. I'm hooked on your program and a definite believer now.

M. Ashton, Brisbane, Australia

Dear Carole:

I have been doing your face exercises for a year now and I just wanted to drop you a line to tell you how glad I am that I found your book. These exercises *really* work. I think I look ten years younger at least.

Terry T., Frankfort, Kentucky

About the author

Carole Maggio is a licensed aesthetician and skincare specialist who has gained wide-ranging attention in the international media. Facercise, developed by Ms. Maggio over twenty years ago, is a widely accepted alternative to cosmetic surgery and has been used for years by celebrities, rock stars, royalty, business leaders and politicians. She is also a bestselling author who has spent decades researching facial exercise techniques and passing them along to her countless thousands of clients worldwide.

Facercise was recently voted one of the top 100 beauty products in the world by *Harpers & Queen* magazine and Ms. Maggio has been called the world's foremost authority on facial exercises. She currently lives in Redondo Beach, California.

For information about Carole Maggio's video and audio tapes, private classes, seminars, her world-renowned skincare brochure or any of her beauty products, you can call 800-597-3555 or 310-540-8048. Her fax number is 310-540-0581. You can also email her at *cmaggio@mminternet.com* or visit the Facebuilder website at facebuilder.com.

Ms. Maggio's postal address is:
Carole Maggio Facercise, Inc.
409 N. Pacific Coast Highway #555
Redondo Beach, CA 90277
USA